The Pyramid Diet

The Pyramid Diet

The Weight is Over!

DANNI LEVY

MICHAEL JOSEPH
an imprint of
PENGUIN BOOKS

MICHAEL JOSEPH

Published by the Penguin Group
Penguin Books Ltd, 80 Strand, London WC2R ORL, England
Penguin Group (USA) Inc., 375 Hudson Street, New York, New York 10014, USA
Penguin Group (Canada), 90 Eglinton Avenue East, Suite 700, Toronto, Ontario, Canada M4P 2Y3
(a division of Pearson Penguin Canada Inc.)
Penguin Ireland, 25 St Stephen's Green, Dublin 2, Ireland (a division of Penguin Books Ltd)
Penguin Group (Australia), 250 Camberwell Road, Camberwell, Victoria 3124, Australia
(a division of Pearson Australia Group Pty Ltd)
Penguin Books India Pvt Ltd, 11 Community Centre, Panchsheel Park, New Delhi – 110 017, India
Penguin Group (NZ), 67 Apollo Drive, Rosedale, Auckland 0632, New Zealand
(a division of Pearson New Zealand Ltd)
Penguin Books (South Africa) (Pty) Ltd, Block D, Rosebank Office Park,
181 Jan Smuts Avenue, Parktown North, Gauteng 2193, South Africa

Penguin Books Ltd, Registered Offices: 80 Strand, London WC2R ORL, England

www.penguin.com

First published 2012
001

Set in 13.5/16pt Garamond MT Std
Typeset by Jouve (UK), Milton Keynes
Printed in Great Britain by Clays Ltd, St Ives plc

A CIP catalogue record for this book is available from the British Library

ISBN: 978-0-718-15895-8

www.greenpenguin.co.uk

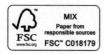

MIX
Paper from
responsible sources
FSC
www.fsc.org   FSC™ C018179

Penguin Books is committed to a sustainable
future for our business, our readers and our planet.
This book is made from Forest Stewardship
Council™ certified paper.

ALWAYS LEARNING   PEARSON

For my husband, Richard – my backbone

Contents

CONTENTS

PART ONE
Introducing the Pyramid Diet

1. The Weight is Over!

If you're reading this, congratulations: you're well on your way to the body you deserve!

First a few words of warning: if you're looking for a quick fix, the Pyramid Diet is not for you. If you believe you have to starve yourself or will always be fat unless you cut out bread and pasta, the Pyramid Diet is not for you. Life presents us with enough ups and downs without having to face the diet rollercoaster too. The Pyramid system is your chance to change your diet for life, so that within a few weeks or months you will never have to worry about losing or gaining weight again.

The unique thing about the Pyramid Diet is that it offers a structured, lifetime approach to food, but one that is flexible. It has the structure we need in all aspects of life, yet it is truly sustainable. In order for something to be sustainable, it needs to be enjoyable, achievable and affordable. The Pyramid is all three of these things.

Introducing the Pyramid Diet

The Pyramid Diet is a rotational eating plan, which offers a structured, lifetime approach to food. It is probably the most balanced diet to date, and works on a principle of varying the amount of carbohydrates we consume every day.

Contrary to popular modern belief, depriving your body of carbohydrates can actually lead to a significant slow-down in your metabolism. So you will learn how to rotate your carbohydrate consumption to keep the metabolism elevated. Your body doesn't have time to adjust to high carbs or low carbs, so it keeps your metabolism working hard to keep up with the changes in your nutritional intake. The Pyramid Diet works, therefore, because it *keeps your body guessing!* It provides you with all the essential macronutrients your body needs, but staggers the intake of carbohydrates to continually stimulate your metabolism and keep it working efficiently.

Carb-cycling is not a new concept. It is something athletes have used to their advantage for many years. I have simply formulated a structure that is easy to understand, easy to follow, and – most importantly – helps you to lose weight and keep it off.

The path you're about to take will see you on the road to sustainable, healthy and proven weight-loss, through a method which can be adapted accordingly once your desired weight is reached.

The Ground Rules

It's All About Carb-Cycling

To begin with, as you will be basing much of your food intake around them, I want to address the ongoing debate surrounding carbohydrates. Followers of popular low- or no-carb diets are led to believe that carbohydrates are the enemy. In truth, they are an essential source of energy and the only form of fuel used by the brain. Severe carb-depletion can lead to fatigue, nausea, mood-swings, breakdown in muscle tissue, weakness, dizziness and bad breath.

If that's not enough to convince you to include a healthy amount of carbs in your diet, you need to know that the majority of weight-loss achieved by cutting carbs is simply water-loss. For every one molecule of glycogen (carbs) our body stores, it stores three molecules of water. So cut the carbs and the water will drain out of your body. Increase your intake again and the water-weight will follow.

On the Pyramid Diet you will have some days on which you can eat carbs and others on which you cannot. Because of the sudden changes in water retention caused by this method, carb-cycling does lead to weight fluctuation. You need to store this information now and accept it, in order to avoid the temptation of banishing carbs altogether in search of a fast 'solution'.

Before you dial the local pizza delivery, I'm afraid to say a meat-feast and chips or a hot dog with onions are not on the menu! Processed carbs such as white bread, doughnuts, white pasta and crisps are strictly forbidden. As you learn more about how the plan works, you'll be glad you banished these ghastly foods to the bin for good.

Now I want to introduce you to the structure of the Pyramid Diet and tell you a little about how it works. It is based on a simple, easy to follow, three-day cycle:

— Day 1: High-carb day
— Day 2: Low-carb day
— Day 3: No-carb day

Think of the Pyramid cycle as a little like interval training on a treadmill. Most of us would prefer to alternate 3 minutes running with 3 minutes walking for half an hour than do

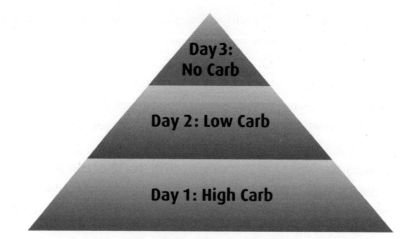

30 minutes solid running. Think of the no-carb day as the sprint, the low-carb day as the jog, and the high-carb day as the walk in the park. Make sense?

Similar methods are often adopted by body-builders and competitive athletes because it allows them to get their bodies to the desired weight or appearance by making simple adjustments to the rotational plan. For simplicity, though, I recommend you stick to the three-day cycle for at least the first three months, or until your desired weight is reached. You may then wish to make amendments to the pattern, which we will discuss in greater detail later on.

And don't worry: while it may appear complex at first, knowing the protein and carb contents of different foods will soon become second nature. Once you've familiarized yourself with them, making choices when you're out and about or on holiday will be much more straightforward than calorie or points counting. And the crucial thing is, so long as you stick to your Pyramid parameters, you will never regain the weight you've lost. It really is as easy as that!

'How much weight can I lose?' I hear you ask. There is no limit to what you can achieve through adopting the Pyramid method, but as a guide you can expect to lose 2–4lbs of fat per week. Note that weight-loss will be fat, not water, as would happen on a purely low-carb approach. What's more, the Pyramid is easy to stick to, as it doesn't deprive you of foods such as bread and pasta.

Having said that, we all like a bit of a challenge when we embark on something new. Whether that something is a new job, new relationship or indeed a new diet, we'd become bored very quickly if things were all plain sailing. So if you're thinking the Pyramid sounds like a piece of cake, fear not, it takes commitment and dedication to stick to the cycle correctly.

GLYCAEMIC INDEX (GI) AND GLYCAEMIC LOAD (GL)

To follow the Pyramid effectively, you'll need to understand about different types of carbohydrates. And to understand these you'll need to understand the terms 'glycaemic index' (GI) and 'glycaemic load' (GL).

The glycaemic index of a carbohydrate is a measure of how quickly it breaks down into glucose, and therefore how quickly the glucose is released into the bloodstream. The quicker it breaks down, the higher the GI for that food. But the GI measure does not take into consideration the quantity of carbohydrate in a meal. The glycaemic load (GL) is based on a food's GI *and* the portion size. There is a standard formula for calculating the GL of a meal or food:

GL = GI × grams of carbohydrate in a serving / 100

We will go into the science in more detail in Chapter 2, but to keep matters simple:

If you follow a low GI and low GL diet, you will lose weight and keep it off more successfully than someone who counts calories but eats high GI foods!

But how do we keep the GL of our meals low on a high-carb day? Well, combining high-carb foods with a source of protein can help to lower the GL of the meal as a whole, and therefore the impact it has on your blood-sugar levels. The lower you can keep the glycaemic load of your meals, the better. Message clear? Excellent! Then I'm confident you can deduce that:

- Foods that are both low GI and low GL will have a small effect on blood-glucose levels, and make excellent dietary choices.
- Foods that have a low GI score but a high GL score are to be avoided. The quantity of the carbohydrate in a typical serving of these foods means they are likely to raise blood-glucose levels quite significantly.
- High GI and low GL foods (such as watermelon) are OK in small quantities, but it is advisable to reduce the GI of these foods by combining them with low GL protein foods. For example, eating watermelon with yoghurt would be better than eating watermelon alone, as it would reduce the total GL of the meal.
- High GI and high GL foods are not permissible on the Pyramid Diet. For this reason, you will not find any of these foods featured in the tables in Part Five. I'm sure you can guess a few of the culprits!

There are three types of foods that are more lethal than

any others when it comes to stalling weight loss. For this reason, they are banned on all three days, including high-carb
day. These are:

- Refined foods such as white bread, pizzas, crisps
  and sugary cereals
- Foods high in saturated fatty acids, like butter,
  cream and full-fat cheese
- Foods that are unashamedly sugary, like sweets, ice
  cream and fizzy drinks

Why You're Sweet Enough Already

Which leads us on to sugar. If you put this devilish substance
into your tea or coffee, stop now! You also need to banish
anything containing added sugars from your kitchen cupboards. Why? Well, table sugar is very high GI and GL and
when we put it into our bodies, the glucose levels in our
blood immediately rise. This prompts the release of insulin
from the pancreas to convert the glucose to glycogen, which
is then utilised in one of three ways:

- 50 per cent is used for immediate energy
- 10 per cent is stored as glycogen in the muscle
  and liver
- 40 per cent is used as fat

This spells bad news for junk foods such as cookies, ice
cream and chocolate bars. You may struggle to cut them out
of your life at first, but the effects on both your health and
physical appearance by making such a small change to your
diet will be well worth the sacrifice.

And the devil-that-is-sugar is also lurking in many unlikely
foods, from ready meals to condiments, yoghurts to so-called

savoury foods such as bread. Unless you're buying something in its natural state, like broccoli or fresh fish, you can never be sure what's been thrown in at the factory. Remember, companies want their products to taste good so you go back for more. All too often this means sugar is added to enhance flavour, so always check the label before buying anything processed to be certain no sugar has been added. This may mean shopping around to find new, acceptable products, but once you've located them you'll find this small change to your diet will really help speed up weight loss.

If you have a sweet tooth and find yourself replacing sugar with artificial sweetener, that's fine, but beware that some sweeteners can have adverse effects on the body too.

MIGUEL SAYS ...

Miguel Toribio-Mateas, the Pyramid Diet's nutritional therapy consultant, says: 'The only sweeteners I'd recommend are xylitol and stevia, which has just become available in the EU. Stevia is a natural product which can be 300 times sweeter than sugar, whilst having zero calories and an almost non-existent effect on blood-sugar levels, so it is great news if you suffer from any degree of insulin resistance.

'Xylitol is a non-fermentable sugar alcohol extracted from fruits and vegetables and fibrous material such as corn husks. It has virtually no aftertaste and provides approximately 40 per cent fewer calories than sucrose. It has a very low glycaemic index: 13, to be precise, compared to glucose, at 100. This means that it elicits a very faint insulin response. There are a variety of foods available containing xylitol, or it can be purchased in powder form as a sweetener.'

In truth, most of the foods which contain sweeteners are foods you should be limiting or eradicating altogether. You've probably heard so many negative things about eating fruit from other popular diets, you're scared half to death to bite into a juicy apple if you want a sweet snack and instead find yourself turning to sweetened, 'diet' candy bars. Relax! The nutrients and fibre in fresh fruit make them ideal for the digestion and utilisation of glucose. What's more, a small piece of fruit only contains around 50 calories. Don't overdose on them, but don't eliminate them.

In Chapter 2 we'll be discussing the science behind the Pyramid and going into greater detail about the never-ending sugar cycle many of us fall into. For now, please be reassured that there are plenty of less fattening alternatives, many of which you will come across on the recipe pages. Once you reach your desired weight, you may want to enjoy the odd sweet treat and that's fine, but you've nothing to lose by opting for healthy alternatives.

Still think low-calorie sweetened foods are less fattening than fruit? Meet Jade.

Miguel and I worked with Jade on the Sky Living TV series *Bigger Than Britney*, which required contestants to follow a strict diet and exercise programme over a period of eight weeks, in a bid to win a lookalike contract. When Jade came to us, she was consuming diet fizzy drinks and candy bars by the shed-load.

Jade recalls: 'I'd always had puppy fat, but during my late teens I started to notice unwelcome weight creeping on around my tummy and thighs. My face didn't really seem to change much, so I could get away with hiding the excess bulge under clothes and most people didn't notice. The problem was, I couldn't hide

JADE'S STORY

it from myself, and I became more and more paranoid about my body.

'I used to stand in front of the mirror trying to find a position which didn't make me look fat, but it was useless. My clothes were beginning to get too tight and before I knew it I was wearing a size 16. Desperate to lose weight, I turned to diet fizzy drinks to fill myself up and replaced mum's home-cooked meals with diet chocolate bars. I didn't eat much at all, and often used to go to bed hungry. I just couldn't understand why I wasn't slimming down when I'd cut back on calories so much! I'd banished bread from my diet and wouldn't touch fruit, because I knew it was sugary, but none of this seemed to make any difference.

'When an opportunity arose to compete in a Britney Spears lookalike challenge *and* lose weight, I couldn't turn it down. That's when I met Danni and Miguel. They explained to me that insulin response is just as crucial as the calorie content of food and drink, and that following a low-calorie diet was not the way to lose weight. I started following the Pyramid Diet and introduced lots of foods back into my life that I thought I'd never have been able to eat if I wanted to slim down.

'Suddenly, I was eating more and losing weight; it was like a dream come true! In eight weeks I went from 12st 2lbs to 10st 7lbs and shrunk from a dress size 16 to a 10–12. I am now able to fit into all my favourite clothes again and no longer feel old and frumpy before my time. Meeting Danni and Miguel was the best thing I ever did. I will never go back to my old way of eating. There is no need, because the Pyramid Diet is so easy to follow and it's more like a way of life in that you are still allowed all the best foods. For me, it was understanding the errors of my ways that opened up the doors to freedom, and I think a lot of people fall into the same trap I did.'

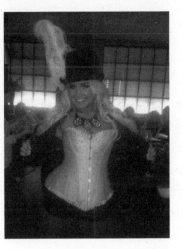
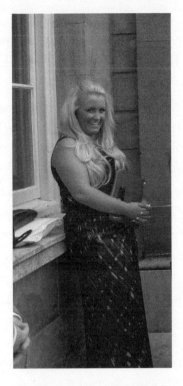

Jade at her heaviest *(left)* Size 10 Jade as Britney Spears *(right)*

Protein and Fat

We established the role of carbs in the Pyramid Diet above; now it's important you also understand the fundamentals of protein and fat intake.

PROTEIN

You may have come across diets that encourage an abnormally high protein intake, or others that involve eating fatty forms of protein in abundance. The Pyramid Diet ensures you consume a substantially beneficial amount of protein daily, whilst also guiding you towards tasty lean sources. Protein is vital for replenishing lost amino acids and building lean muscle tissue. It also stimulates the release of glucagon, which is a fat-burning hormone. There are dozens of choices when it comes to ensuring you're eating enough protein and these don't have to be foods containing undesirable types of fats.

On the Pyramid Diet you should aim to consume around 1g of protein per lb of body-weight. This goal applies every day, including high-carb days. This protein intake is most effective when eaten throughout the day, preferably at each meal. For example, you will not reap maximum benefit from enjoying just oats for breakfast, followed by a piece of fruit and soup for lunch. It is advisable to divide your protein intake equally between all six meals to ensure you are getting enough. If you miss out on protein at breakfast, make sure you get a good helping of amino acids mid-morning, especially if you've been rushing to work or paid a visit to the gym. This will ensure your body preserves lean muscle mass, which is the last thing you want to be burning for energy.

FAT

Fat is yet another topic of great debate and recent claims will probably have left you confused. Advocates of certain high-fat diets will tell you saturated fat has now been shown not to increase your risk of heart disease unless it's eaten in conjunction with a high-carbohydrate diet. But experts are unsure whether this is because individuals who have a tendency to opt for fatty foods also eat lots of starchy carbs, such as white bread and pasta. Many high-carb dishes such as pizza and burgers are also extremely high in saturated fat.

The bottom line is that saturated fat is saturated fat. Overdose on it and it will clog up your arteries, leading to all manner of health problems.

Diets that are extremely low in fat can be equally damaging to your body. Fat is an essential part of our daily food consumption and an excellent form of energy. Just because you're eating something with a high fat content does not mean your body will automatically store this as fat. The Pyramid Diet will help you to choose foods containing the most beneficial sorts of fat and help you decide when you should be eating them.

Although the Pyramid Diet does not count calories or require you to limit your fat intake as such, you nevertheless need to be aware that fat is the most calorie-dense macronutrient: 1g of fat contains 9 calories, whilst 1g of protein or carbohydrate contains only 4. So whilst foods like natural peanut butter feature in the list of recommended fats, be energy savvy and avoid eating it by the spoon. Realistically speaking, you need to create a deficit of a whopping 3,500 calories to lose just 1lb of body-weight, so please keep this in mind. The Pyramid will help your body to metabolize energy efficiently, but there is not a diet in the world that can wave a magic wand and make excess calories disappear from your digestive system.

Cut Out the Salt

It is often the case that fatty fast foods are high in salt. Not only does excess salt contribute to high blood pressure and heart problems, it also contributes to fluid retention. So although calorie-free in itself, piling on the salt often means piling on the pounds.

The Water of Life

It is imperative that you drink a minimum of 8 glasses of water a day to avoid dehydration and enable your body to metabolize fats effectively. Exact requirements will vary according to your height, weight and physical output, but rest assured you'll struggle to drink too much.

If you're bored of hearing this, perhaps you'd like to hear the benefits of adequate fluid intake. Well, it's not uncommon to think you're hungry when actually it's thirst your body is suffering from, so drink a glass of water before each meal to prevent over-eating. Also, when it comes to shedding water-weight (which can cause huge differences in visual appearance), you actually need to be drinking *more* water in order to force your body to let go of any excess fluid. Think of your body as being like a camel storing water in its humps for those long treks across the desert (and who wants to look like a camel?!). If you don't put water into your system, your body will hold on to any fluid for dear life, as it's scared of becoming dehydrated.

If you drink black or green tea, you may count this towards your quota, but you should still be drinking plain and simple water on a day-to-day basis. You may try adding a squeeze of fresh lemon but do not add sugary, concentrated cordials.

Alcohol

There is no easy answer here: the lower your alcohol intake, the easier it will be to lose weight. Alcohol contains 7 calories per gram and these calories will be burned first by your body. So calories from fat and glucose will not be used up by your body until the energy from the alcohol has been burned off.

It doesn't take a rocket scientist to work out that the fat and glucose may well end up being stored as fat. I will cover this topic in more detail in Chapter 5, but for now you'll need to accept that drinking and weight-loss do not go hand in hand.

To Recap: Notes for Your Fridge

- Carbohydrates will be consumed as part of the cycle in order to make the most of your body's metabolic abilities.
- Protein is a vital part of your daily diet and *must* be consumed throughout the day.
- Fats are essential, but choose the right ones.
- Any foods containing added sugar are strictly prohibited.
- Drink water to shed water-weight.

2. Why the Pyramid Diet?

If you're a serial dieter, you may well be asking yourself why you should embark on the Pyramid Diet when so many other diets have failed to fulfil their promises. Headlines like 'Achieve instant results', 'Get a flat stomach in 14 days' and 'Lose 10lbs of belly fat per week' flood the media and continue to lure us into their trap.

By far the biggest step towards achieving weight-loss on any programme is commitment and dedication, and you cannot possibly be committed if you don't have faith in what you are being asked to do. Before signing on the dotted line, you'll almost certainly want to read real success stories, be assured the programme is scientifically sound, and, most importantly, have an understanding of why the Pyramid works.

You'll appreciate by now that the Pyramid Diet is based on a continuous three-day cycle. So, whilst most modern diets start at the beginning and finish at the end, you are going to need to get used to working an entirely new shift pattern.

Step Away From the Yo-Yo!

Dieting has always reminded me of a game show. You know the kind, where the glittering, over-enthusiastic host announces to the players: 'You've won the cash, now can you keep it?!' Most of us are capable of losing weight. Whether it's a few pounds, a dress size or even a stone or more, we are great at charging out of the blocks full of intent and conviction. Some of us make it over the first hurdle, which is normally some kind of no-carb, low-calorie or almost-starvation phase, then decide we've suffered enough and slow back down to a nice comfortable walk. Some of us make it past the second hurdle, full of new-found confidence as a result of instant 'weight-loss' experienced in the first week or two, and continue to follow the plan to the letter. But then there comes a time we crave a bowl of pasta or a social meal arises, and the forthcoming hurdle is simply impossible to jump. So, we forgive ourselves for our sins with the intention of returning to the diet the following day. In reality, though, once we stray from the yellow-brick road, it's game over!

'Aww, I'm so sorry, wasn't she a brilliant contestant though?!' says the game-show host to a sympathetic audience. He then turns back to the disheartened player: 'You couldn't keep your cash, but have you had a nice time?' Of course you haven't had a nice time – you'd built up so much hope! The cash was in the bag! But despite having won it fair and square it is cruelly taken away from you.

That, my friends, is the tale of the 'dietary journey'. But the word 'diet' simply means 'the usual food and drink of an animal or person'. So why should a diet start at the beginning and end at the end? This all too familiar journey leaves us in limbo once we cross the finish line, and all that unwanted weight we thought we'd waved goodbye to soon comes right back.

The diagram overleaf illustrates a typical modern diet. These diets normally start off being very restrictive to ensure you lose weight. They then allow you to reintroduce certain foods into your life, but only at a level that will not allow those unwanted pounds to creep back on. So far, so good. Then you reach the final stage, in which you are expected to maintain the diet for the rest of your life, having had a huge carrot dangled right in front of your nose in the intermediary stage. One 'harmless' chocolate bar a week becomes a chocolate bar a day and, hey presto, you've fallen off the end of the linear diet track. So what do you do? You go right back to the beginning and start again! I hope that now you can see the flaws of this method diagrammatically, you will appreciate it wasn't you making the mistakes. If the earth was flat we'd fall off the end, right? If you've tried these diets and felt as if you 'failed', you didn't. You simply came to the end of the path.

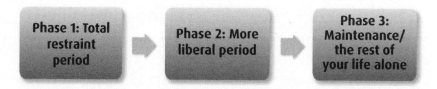

The Pyramid Diet is not open-ended like that linear dietary racetrack from your past. Instead, the Pyramid Diet goes round and round. And once you've constructed your circle you'll be able to treat it as your own circle of life, with the necessary foods and beverages for a satisfying, slender way of living. The Pyramid is a diet for life itself, which allows you to take everything in your stride and not race for the finish line, continually running out of puff.

The diagram opposite illustrates the cyclical pattern created by the Pyramid Diet. You will see there are no loose ends, no start and finish point and no way you can fall off. The Pyramid never leaves you to fend for yourself in the tempting world of food. It guides you through thick and thin and helps you to negotiate obstacles along the way.

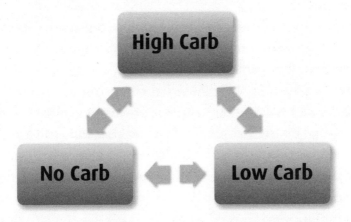

In order to help you better understand why the Pyramid works so well, it is useful to identify the good reasons why so many other diets are doomed to disaster.

Diet Disaster No. 1: Phantom Weight-Loss

You step on the scales after just a few short days of dieting and they say you've lost 5 lbs. So that's how much you've lost, right? Wrong! Well, most of the time anyway. Many recent popular diets are based on a low-carb approach, eliminating this macronutrient almost entirely. This is significant because, as a reminder, for every one molecule of glycogen (carbohydrates) your body holds, it also holds three molecules of water. Unfortunately, your everyday bathroom scales do not differentiate between water and fat, and it's not unusual for water retention to tip the needle 3, 4 or even 5 lbs over the 'true' reading. But of course when we start a low- or no-carb diet, the excess water is flushed from our systems. This leads to a welcome boost at the first weigh-in, but will only last as long as you stay off the carbs completely. Just one bowl of oats or slice of bread will send you crashing back down to planet earth.

If that's not enough to convince you, remember it takes a deficit of a whopping 3,500 calories to lose just 1lb – that's almost two days' worth of food for the average person.

This is why it is recommended when following the Pyramid Diet that you only compare your weight against previous readings taken on the same type of day because you are likely to be at least 2–3lbs heavier on high-carb days than low-carb days, as your body will be holding more water. If you choose to weigh yourself on no-carb days, it is imperative you resist the temptation to start cutting carbohydrates out of your life in the belief you will reach your goal weight faster. This is simply not true.

Furthermore, no-carb diets come with some hefty downsides.

- They are not sustainable. Eating out, social occasions and even home cooking is extremely limited for those on a daily no-carb eating plan. The majority of followers stray from such programmes after just a few short days or weeks as a result.
- They are unforgiving. Stray from the path for just one meal and those dreaded scales (which up until now have been your best friend) will turn against you and insist you have gained weight instantly.
- They can lead to side-effects such as fatigue, nausea, bad breath, weakness and mood-swings.

Diet Disaster No. 2: Calorie Counting

Whilst calorie counting is an effective way of measuring the amount of fuel needed by the body, many dieters get caught up in obsessive calorie counting or restricting their intake too harshly. This sends the body into starvation mode, reducing the amount of energy it needs to function and slowing the metabolic rate. What's more, calories from different forms of nutrition are metabolized in different ways and this has to be taken into consideration when composing an eating plan.

Many calorie-counting dieters live on the verge of starvation, relying on soups and shakes for nutrition. Not only will this make it very hard to keep their weight down in future, but their brain function, energy levels, skin tone and social life will also suffer. As soon as they resume normal eating patterns, the body will naturally hang on to every last bit of energy for dear life and store it as fat in case it is starved again in the weeks to come. Sadly, for many dieters this leads to a vicious cycle which can last a lifetime.

If you're serious about losing weight and keeping it off, resist the temptation to count calories and rest assured that the unique system the Pyramid Diet offers will ensure you do not eat too much.

Diet Disaster No. 3: Meals on Wheels

And when we're not sure how much food to put on our plates, there is always Diet Disaster No. 3. This latest media-plugged offering even takes care of the cooking for you. Let's face it, our modern lifestyles and professional commitments can often make home-cooked meals a challenge. But fear not, there is a solution: the meals-on-wheels service – or at least that's what some diet companies will tell you.

Credit where credit's due, there are companies who produce good-quality, well-balanced, nutritious meals delivered to your door. They do the calorie counting for you and ensure that you are eating a healthy, balanced diet to aid weight-loss. They even provide a counselling service to help you stay on the straight and narrow. All you have to do is pop your meals in the microwave, sit back and watch the pounds fall off! So what could possibly go wrong?

Many subscribers of home-delivered meal services claim the portions are too small to leave them feeling truly satisfied, and whilst the food they provide normally tastes great, most of us end up resenting the weight-loss process if we're left feeling hungry. The cost of these programmes is also an issue, forcing some of us to abandon our quest before we've reached the finish line. For those of us who successfully lose the desired amount of weight, once we feel ready to return to normality, we're left with the challenge of trying to replicate similar meals at home in order to ensure the weight stays off. Of course, without a personal chef to prepare our food and weigh every single morsel that passes our lips, this is a task most of us just cannot pull off. Those extra pounds we thought we'd waved goodbye to soon start piling their way back on to our waistlines and the dreaded diet cycle starts all over again.

So there we have it: three of the most common diet disasters. If you've already fallen for their charms and since regained the weight you lost in those first few tough days or weeks, you owe it to yourself to switch to a balanced and sustainable approach that won't leave you dangling above thin ice at the end of your dietary 'journey'.

One girl who certainly did succumb to the ideals of 'meals on wheels' was 30-year-old Nicole Alger, another *Bigger Than Britney* contestant. Nicole came to us desperate to lose weight after her busy lifestyle as a working mum led her to sign up to a meals-on-wheels diet service which promised results.

Nicole says: 'I'd pretty much tried every trick in the book, from starving myself, to carb-free diets, to bars and shakes. I'd never managed to regain my old figure after childbirth and longed to fit into a size 10 again. An advertisement came on one evening when I'd just sat down to a low-calorie ready-meal, for a service that literally prepared and delivered suitable slimmer's meals to your plate, saving you the confusing task of choosing what to eat and avoiding the potential pitfall of consuming too much in one sitting. It had to be worth a go, so I signed up there and then!

'The meals provided by the service were pretty tasty, but they didn't fill me up. In fact, I'd say I was hungrier after dinner than I was before! Because I knew they were low-calorie, I'd then allow myself a sneaky snack of cheese crackers or a bag of crisps to help "fill the hole" left after my main meal. Not only that, I found I was spending a lot more money on the plan than I was before. Being a mum with a family to feed, I was having to buy all the normal food shopping anyway, so the cost of my meals came in on top of this.

'After six weeks on the plan, I hadn't lost a single ounce and I was beginning to resent not being able to eat the same foods as my family and friends at mealtimes. I gave it up and shortly afterwards I met Danni and Miguel, who introduced me to the Pyramid Diet and, incredibly, allowed me to lead a "normal" dietary life again. In just eight weeks, I achieved my goal of "being in the 9s", and went from a dress size 16 to a perfect 10. The best part for me was losing 5 inches from my waist, as up until that point I'd always felt a little like I was still pregnant! I am finally able to go out wearing strappy tops without having to worry about bingo wings, and enjoy eating "normal" foods with the rest of the family. I have really embraced the cooking side of things too, and enjoy trying new and exciting Pyramid recipes when I get the time. The desserts are all family favourites!'

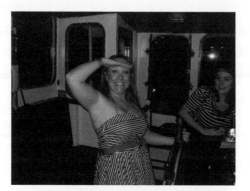

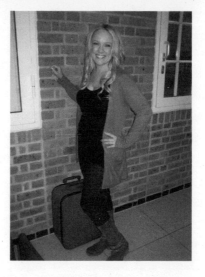

(top) Nicole at size 14–16
(bottom) A much slimmer, happier Nicole

Whilst it would not be fair to say the above methods lead to disaster for everyone (in fact, for the brave, bold and determined among us, they may lead to great success), I feel it's time we studied the science behind an alternative method fit for a lifetime: the Pyramid Diet.

The Science

Carb-Cycling: Your Friend for Life

We've heard how the Pyramid Diet works because it *keeps your body guessing*. Whilst consuming more calories than we need leads to weight gain, it is important to recognize that calories derived from different macronutrients are utilized by the body in different ways. Each major food group triggers a different type of chemical breakdown in the body. For these reasons, when it comes to sculpting our bodies into pillars of perfection, we can't just sit back with a calculator and call a calorie a calorie. The composition of each calorie we consume is just as relevant as its energy content.

That is why eliminating certain food groups altogether is not advisable if you are seeking long-term, sustainable weight-loss. In order to develop a toned and shapely body, of course you will need to burn fat, but you'll also need to build lean muscle. I'm not talking bulging biceps and killer quads, I'm talking about a process called 'anabolism'. To help you better understand anabolism and the importance of carbohydrates in stimulating this metabolic process, let's first take a look at how our metabolisms function.

The term 'metabolism' is something most of us are familiar with. We know we want to speed it up and we know those blessed with fast metabolisms tend to find it easy to stay in shape. But why is this? What exactly is our metabolism and how does it influence our body shape? Well, the word metabolism refers to the set of chemical reactions that happen inside our bodies in order to maintain life. These chemical reactions determine whether we store or break down fat and build or lose muscle. There are two different pathways the metabolism can take in order to stimulate changes to the composition of our bodies: anabolism and catabolism.

Anabolism is the process by which muscle is constructed. It is the building of protein needed to create muscle growth. In order for your metabolism to be anabolic, you need to be in positive calorie balance, which means consuming more calories than your body needs. Naturally, you will be concerned that instigating anabolism means you will store more fat; you're right! Unfortunately, protein synthesis (or muscle building) is something that cannot take place without some excess food being stored as fat. That is why body-builders tend to 'bulk up' before dieting down for competitions. It would be impossible to build lean muscle alone without packing on an ounce of fat.

OK, so you're not a body-builder, you don't want to be muscular and you definitely don't want to gain fat, so why on earth should you be concerned with anabolism? You'll be pleased to know the explanation behind this conundrum is neither tedious nor complex. To explain how the Pyramid Diet keeps your body guessing, I must tell you about the metabolism's counteracting process: catabolism.

Catabolism is the process by which your body burns fat, and occurs when you are in negative calorie balance and therefore need to draw on your body's stored energy reserves to function. Whilst going catabolic sounds like the obvious choice for those wanting to lose weight, if your body were to be in a catabolic state for a prolonged period of time, you'd be forcing your system into continuous negative calorie balance, which in turn would cause a metabolic slow down. This has a detrimental effect on weight-loss and puts the brakes on the slimming process. We can only withstand a catabolic state for so long before clinging on to those precious fat reserves for dear life. Our bodies become so scared they won't receive their next meal, that instead of revving up the metabolism to burn fat, they slow it right down to preserve all they can.

Go anabolic, though, and yes, you've guessed it, we fire up our metabolisms and ensure that on low- and no-carb days, when we do go catabolic, there is no danger of clinging on to fat stores. If that's not enough to convince you to go anabolic every third day, spending prolonged periods in a catabolic state will lead to lack of libido, wrinkles and possibly even joint pain and hair loss. What's more, as we age, catabolism begins to dominate over anabolism, so periodically sending your body into an anabolic state will allow for tissue rejuvenation and help to slow that dreaded ageing process. (Exercise is also an important factor in boosting the levels of anabolic hormones we produce, and we will discuss this in some detail in Chapter 13.)

Whilst Pyramid dieters are discouraged from counting their daily calorie intake, naturally you will consume fewer calories on low- and no-carb days than you will on high-carb days. The desire for carbohydrates you will experience on these high-carb days will ensure your body is in an anabolic state every third day without you even thinking about it. Similarly, cutting down on your carbohydrate consumption on low- and no-carb days will send your system straight into catabolism, drawing upon your fat reserves because your glycogen (carb) stores are depleted and, at least on no-carb days, putting you in negative calorie balance.

The carb-cycling method is the only dietary system which makes use of this clever trickery. Your body just can't guess your next move, so it keeps on building muscle and burning fat; the ultimate recipe for lean loveliness. This is what low-calorie, low-carb and many other popular diets fail to recognize. We are designed to be predators forced to hunt down our meals. Thousands of years ago we weren't tempted by over-loaded plates and tempting treats, but were left to forage for food and be grateful for every last mouthful. Our bodies are therefore designed to protect and preserve anything we put into them. Once we recognize this, does it not become obvious that depriving ourselves of energy, vitamins and minerals and certain food groups is not going to keep the weight off long-term? Of course it does!

Get Your Daily Protein!

So you're clued up on the science behind carb-cycling. But rotating your carbohydrate consumption alone will not necessarily lead to successful weight loss. Think of the Pyramid Diet as being like a jigsaw puzzle. There are many components to it which all have to slot into place if maximum benefits are to be reaped. The second component I'd like to tell you about is the recommended daily protein intake. As briefly mentioned in Chapter 1, this is 1g of protein per lb of body weight. So, for example, if you weigh 150lbs, you should aim to consume a minimum of 150g of protein each day in relatively equal portions throughout the day, preferably at each meal. This would equate to 25g of protein per sitting. (You will find the carb, protein and fat contents of popular Pyramid foods in Part Five.)

Failing to consume adequate protein will almost certainly be detrimental to your progress. Protein is not just for body-builders and competitive athletes. Increasing your intake will not turn you into the Incredible Hulk. Accepting this now will allow you to enjoy the many positive effects sufficient protein will have on your body. Once you begin to experience these physical changes for yourself, you will never question this component of the diet again.

So how can simply consuming more of a certain food group have maximum benefits for your body? First, high-protein foods not only make you feel full for longer, they also stabilize blood-sugar levels, avoiding sugar spikes caused by carbohydrate intake. This in turn reduces the cravings you feel for sugary sweets and snacks. Not only that, protein actually helps to speed up your metabolism. This makes it the perfect macronutrient for complementing the tug of war between anabolism and catabolism created by the Pyramid method.

LESS WEIGHT FOR YOUR PLATE

But there are yet more benefits to proteins. You may remember that protein comes with an energy 'price tag' of 4 calories per gram. This makes it apparently equal to carbohydrates, but as you may suspect, things are not quite as simple when it comes to totting up the treats. As far as proteins are concerned, we need only add around 70 per cent of their calorific content to our total. So, for example, if you ate a six-egg-white omelette, a form of pure protein totalling 100 calories, you'd only have provided your body with around 70 calories of energy by the time you'd digested them. This is because a protein's thermic effect (the amount of energy required to digest and absorb it) stands at a whopping 30 per cent. By contrast, the thermic effect of carbohydrates is only 7–8 per cent, and fats 2–3 per cent, as they are processed and turned into body fat more easily than any other food group. Subsequently, not only do you save on calories when consuming high-protein foods, they also lead to a higher metabolic rate and therefore greater fat loss.

EAT PROTEIN TO BURN FAT

The benefits of protein don't end there. When we eat protein foods, it stimulates the production of glucagon, a hormone that opposes insulin. Glucagon actually shifts the body's focus towards burning stored fat and carbohydrates for energy. Both insulin and glucagon are secreted by the pancreas, but whereas insulin works to lower blood-sugar levels, glucagon does the opposite. You may recall from the opening chapter how the release of insulin into the bloodstream can spell bad news for your waistline. Glucagon helps to counteract the effects of insulin by causing the liver to convert glycogen into glucose and release it into the bloodstream. Put simply, glucagon helps you burn more fat, a great reason to ensure you don't neglect the daily recommended protein intake dictated by the Pyramid Diet.

You may have heard claims that high protein equals high fat and therefore an increased risk of heart disease. Relax. The Pyramid Diet ensures you consume a combination of both plant- and animal-based proteins which have only positive effects on both weight-loss and long-term well being. There are good and bad choices within any given food group, and you'll be encouraged to opt for lean sources of protein as opposed to highly processed meats containing all the wrong fats. And even if you're not a vegetarian, have a look at Chapter 10 to find lots of alternatives to meat.

The Right Carbs

If you want to lose fat and keep it off for a lifetime, it is my duty to remind you that all foods containing added sugar belong in the bin and should never slime their way on to your shelves again.

Remember in the opening chapter we saw how sugar triggers the release of insulin from the pancreas? This is not something to be taken lightly. The repeated insulin injection can be very damaging. 'Insulin resistance', 'Syndrome X', 'glucose intolerance', 'prediabetes' and 'metabolic syndrome' are all terms used to describe the dangerous sugar trap so many of us fall foul of. It can firmly implant its claws into your brain and plunge you into a rapidly descending medical spiral, from which only the well informed can make an escape. For the purpose of this book and to avoid confusion, I will hereafter refer to this condition as metabolic syndrome.

The term metabolic syndrome dates as far back as the 1950s, but came into common usage in the late 1970s. It has since become a key factor in the understanding of human metabolism. Today, we fight a growing epidemic of obesity, diabetes and cardiovascular disease, often linked to patients having slowly developed metabolic syndrome over a period of years. Whilst I don't seek to baffle you with science beyond your interests, I am of the firm belief it is vital to learn the causes of metabolic syndrome if you are to achieve your ideal body weight. Staying out of the danger zone will make losing weight and keeping it off a whole lot easier. So what exactly is metabolic syndrome, what causes it and how can you prevent or even reverse it?

As we briefly talked about in Chapter 1, when you put sugar (or glucose) into your body, the pancreas releases insulin, which transports the glucose from the blood to the cells. If the glucose is not needed for energy, it is converted into glycogen and either stored in the liver and muscle (only around 10 per cent) or stored as fat around the body (around 40 per cent). This glucose is then either burned for energy or stored as fat. The rate at which the pancreas springs into action depends on how rapidly the food you have just eaten is digested into the bloodstream. Processed carbohydrates devoid of fibre, such as bleached white products, are rapidly digested and quickly converted to glucose by the body. Eating these types of foods therefore causes the pancreas to release insulin quickly, in order to lower your glucose levels. Whilst many people are fortunate enough to be able to withstand this type of diet for years, others are not so lucky. The outcome of an overworked pancreas, forced to inject insulin in such urgent and successive bursts, can be devastating.

Once metabolic syndrome gets hold of you, successfully losing weight can seem like an endless uphill battle; that is unless you give yourself a reality check and take action against sugar. And when I say action, I mean business! If you're thinking you can simply rid your cupboards of the sugars you can see, then think again. As I've said already, sugar slimes its way into all sorts of unlikely products and often manages to hide away unnoticed. Sneaky manufacturers use enough alternative terms for sugar to compile an entirely new foreign language! Whilst I could write you a list as long as my arm, below are the most common terms printed on food labels to disguise the sugar lurking inside.

The Sugar Alphabet

– Barley malt
– Cane sugar
– Concentrated fruit juice
– Corn fructose
– Corn sweetener
– Corn syrup
– Demerara sugar
– Dextrin
– Dextrose
– Diatase
– Fructose
– Galactose
– Glucose
– Grape sugar
– Hydrolysed starch
– Maltodextrin
– Maltose
– Manitol
– Malt syrup
– Maple syrup
– Polydextrose
– Sorbitol
– Sucrose

You may find it useful to copy this list and take it with you to the supermarket. You'll be surprised what an obstacle course shopping becomes when trying to navigate your way around these terms. Once you become familiar with them, they'll stick out like a sore thumb and you'll soon be steering well clear of anything that sounds as if it's going to hang around your midriff for dear life.

Another important point to be made when doing the weekly shop is that ingredients are always listed in order of weight, so the main ingredients in the packaged food always come first. With this in mind, take a look through those snacks you stack your shelves with in the belief they're the healthy option. Do any of the terms from the sugar alphabet feature high up on the ingredients lists? Thought so! There's only one place for these sweet treats, and that's the bin.

Surprisingly, foods we think of as dessert items are not always the worst culprits. For example, a Krispy Kreme original glazed doughnut contains 10g of sugar, whilst a Yoplait Original strawberry yoghurt, which grabs our attention with its '99% fat free' label, contains a whopping 26g of sugar. (If I had a pound for every one of you who'd bet on the yoghurt being the lower sugar option, I certainly would never be playing the lottery again!) The lesson to be learned is that even the 'foodies' among us sometimes jump to the wrong conclusion. Unless you're 100 per cent sure what you're about to put into your mouth, always remember these words:

Read Before You Feed!

Oh, and before you dash out to shop for doughnuts, I'm afraid these are a form of refined carbohydrates that have no place in the lives of Pyramid followers. Why not? Well, when we consume processed or refined foods such as white bread or sweet cereals, all of the ingested sugar quickly rushes to the bloodstream. This gives us a 'sugar rush', providing us with a quick, short-lived surge of energy, but our bodies promptly react by calling on the pancreas to produce insulin to remove this excess sugar from the bloodstream. As a result, you then have significantly lower blood sugar. For those of you who haven't already guessed where this is leading, that almost euphoric feeling you experienced just a few minutes earlier will now have disappeared, resulting in a craving for more sugar. At this moment, which I call the 'carb comedown', we are incredibly susceptible to hitting the biscuit tin, thus initiating the infamous sugar cycle.

Once we fall into the sugar trap, we're little more than a hamster on a wheel, and it becomes extremely difficult to escape the cycle. Our bodies start releasing more and more insulin from the pancreas to combat all that glucose we're putting into our systems. But the more regularly and aggressively we pump insulin into our systems, the more the body begins to resist its effects and the closer we become to developing metabolic syndrome.

The Pyramid Diet is designed to guide you away from the blood-sugar battlefield and into calmer seas, where sugar cravings, unwanted weight-gain and demanding diets are a thing of the past.

For further clarity, you may find it useful to read the table overleaf, which illustrates the way in which certain foods impact on our blood-sugar levels – and, in turn, the release of insulin – using the glycaemic index (GI). As we've already heard, low GI foods cause a slow and steady rise in blood-sugar levels and help to delay feelings of hunger. High GI foods, on the other hand, are foods which are known to cause a dramatic and sudden increase in blood-sugar levels. These types of foods should be avoided as much as possible, even on high-carb days. You will find more details in the tables in Part Five. Use them to help you find low GI alternatives to your favourite foods, whether dining out or eating in.

High GI

- White bread
- White pitta bread
- Pretzels
- Cornflakes
- White rice
- Potato
- Chicken burger
- Cod in batter
- Chicken and mushroom pie
- Watermelon

Low GI

- Granary bread
- Wholewheat tortillas
- Popcorn (unsweetened)
- Porridge (unsweetened)
- Wholewheat pasta
- Chicken drumsticks (uncoated)
- Grilled cod
- Chicken chasseur
- Sweet potato

As you will be well aware by now, the Pyramid Diet does not eliminate carbs from the kitchen. Cutting out an entire food group is neither physically nor psychologically beneficial. Not only that, carbohydrates are a crucial cog in the Pyramid wheel. The emphasis therefore should be on choosing the right carbohydrates, containing only natural sugars and plenty of fibre.

Low GI carbohydrate-rich foods provide slow-burning

energy, perfect prior to a workout. They are also the number-one food chosen by your brain. Found predominantly on Day 1 of the Pyramid Diet, they provide a long-lasting sense of fullness and add substantial bulk to our dinner plates. These types of foods are normally less pricey than protein foods, and when rich in fibre they ensure our digestive systems keep functioning smoothly.

Train Your Brain

Now that you know how the Pyramid Diet works on your body, it's time to focus on the mind. The mental aspect of dieting is often overlooked, but is vitally important if you are to achieve and maintain your goals. Fortunately, there is a solution to that constant battle between body and brain which you may well have experienced on past diets.

YOU DON'T BELONG TO YOUR BODY: YOUR BODY BELONGS TO YOU!

The final component that makes the Pyramid Diet so successful is sustainability. Any lifetime approach to food must be both mentally and physiologically rewarding. If you allow your body to become too familiar with certain eating patterns, it will learn to protect and preserve the energy you consume in line with its paleolithic make-up. This is to say, your metabolism will tick along its merry way, slowly but surely storing any excess food it can get its hands on in case of a rainy day. Any diet which requires the follower to settle into a constant way of eating will inevitably have limited sustainability. Once your body becomes accustomed to your new tricks, it's game over for weight-loss. I'll say it again, the

Pyramid Diet is one of very few systems to keep your body guessing; day after day, week after week, year after year.

Quick-fix diets have a tendency to make us feel as if food rules our lives. After a few delirious days of deprivation, almost every object around us appears to resemble our favourite cake or preferred comfort meal which we simply cannot have. Instead, we are restricted to soups, shakes or turkey slices in a bid to shift the bulge at lightning speed. Allowing your body to rule over your brain is a recipe for life-long weight fluctuation. There is only so long one can adhere to such an unnatural programme for, after a while, those hard-fought pounds you lost will slowly but surely creep back on. The problem is that our brains don't think rationally when it comes to food either. They tell us to eat every tasty treat in sight and deal with the consequences later. This is why we turn to fad diets to do the thinking for us. So what's the solution?

HOW TO TRAIN YOUR BRAIN

If you want to take control of your weight, it's time to train your brain into making rational and balanced food choices. Your body and brain will then start to work in harmony with one another, possibly for the first time in your adult life. Once this happens the battle with the bulge is finally over, enabling you to be at peace with both your diet and your physical appearance.

The more determined among us soldier on along the starvation route, determined that the messages the brain sends to the body can be safely ignored in aid of faster weight-loss. Research reveals quite the opposite. Whilst gorging ourselves on anything that takes our fancy is definitely not conducive to a healthy waistline, depriving the body to the point of mental and emotional stress can actually cause weight-*gain*.

The main culprit responsible for stress-related weight-gain, especially around the midriff, is a hormone called cortisol. This is secreted in response to stress, which very often comes about as a result of harsh dieting. Studies have shown that people who yo-yo diet in a way which restricts their food intake have higher levels of cortisol. Most research points specifically to serial dieters becoming 'apple shaped', eventually storing the majority of excess fat around their waists, in line with elevated cortisol levels. This accumulation of abdominal fat is typically very difficult to shift.

The Pyramid Diet works against elevated cortisol levels and helps keep stress levels low. Good-quality, high-protein foods, low GI carbohydrates and healthy fats, all fundamental parts of the Pyramid, are foods known to lower cortisol levels. The phytonutrients and vitamins present in fresh fruit and vegetables can inhibit cortisol production too. (You'll learn more about the necessary inclusion of fruits and vegetables on the Pyramid Diet in Part Two.) Sugar-laden refined carbs and high GI foods have the reverse effect, causing the body's cortisol levels to rise. You needn't worry when following the Pyramid plan, though, as you'll be gently guided away from these foods, and, best of all, you won't miss them!

The Science Made Simple

- Fad diets are to be avoided, and must not be used in conjunction with (in whole or in part) the Pyramid Diet
- Carb-cycling keeps the metabolism ticking

- Protein intake is fundamental to fat-burning and weight-loss
- Processed foods and products containing added sugar inhibit fat-burning
- The Pyramid Diet will help you to strike up a good relationship between your body and your brain

Now it's up to you to construct your very own Pyramid from the foods *you* enjoy. The Pyramid Diet is not about packaged meals or shakes; it is about eating real food in real social situations. All you need to do is identify the foods you can and can't eat, and choose from the ones you love the most. This is where Part Two comes in: 'Building the Foundations'. Shall we go there now? Follow me!

PART TWO
Building the Foundations

3. The Great Carb Debate

Whilst the Pyramid Diet does not eliminate any of the major food groups, there are certain foods best avoided. If you're ready to say hello to the body you deserve, you'll also need to be prepared to wave goodbye to a few old friends from your dietary past.

The Great Carb Debate

Sit back, take a deep breath and be prepared for a discussion we could continue for centuries. (We won't, of course – I aim to make this as painless and straightforward as possible!) As you already know, choosing the right carbs is just as important as sticking to the maximum carb intake on any given day. You've binned the white starchy bread, ditched the sugar and prohibited the processed junk, but which carbohydrate foods can actually help, not hinder, your progress?

As you know, the most important factors to take into account where carbs are concerned are the glycaemic index and glycaemic load, which we spoke about in Part One. The GL for each food gives us a more accurate assessment based on how much carbohydrate is in a serving. So, for example, the carbohydrate in watermelon is high GI, but there isn't much of it, making the overall glycaemic load relatively low. On the flip-side, raisins have a medium GI, but a high GL.

The Pyramid prohibits both high GI and high GL foods. You will be able to enjoy the types of carbohydrate foods that trigger a slow rise in blood-sugar levels, but not those which cause a fast insulin spike. If you're unsure whether it's acceptable to consume a certain type of food, *read before you feed* and check the tables in Part Five.

It is occasionally possible to reduce the damage by combining high GI/GL foods with low ones. For example, raisins are medium GI and high GL, but throwing a handful of low GI cashew nuts into the mix would bring the total glycaemic load of this snack down considerably. So you can enjoy raisins *if* you combine them with nuts. However, you will only be allowed to do this with a very small number of foods, as the vast majority of high GI/GL foods are not allowed. If a high GI/GL food is 'Pyramid-Approved' in Part Five, you must apply this 'mixing' method to make it truly acceptable, and only enjoy it in moderation.

The following are examples of potentially high GI/GL meals and snacks being brought down to a safe level by including low-GI foods in the dish. The easiest way to achieve this is to add protein:

- Wholewheat spaghetti with bolognese sauce
- Brown rice with egg (egg-fried rice) and chicken
- Watermelon with low-fat Greek yoghurt
- Raisins with cashew nuts

Carbs Aren't Always Complex!

The glycaemic index is not the only determining factor where carbs are concerned. Carbohydrate foods fall into two categories: simple and complex. It is perfectly fine to consume both types, but certain foods from each group should be avoided, whilst others are Pyramid-worthy choices.

SIMPLE CARBOHYDRATES

Simple carbohydrates are essentially sugars, and both natural and refined sugars fall into this category. We spoke about these in depth in Chapter 2, so I am confident you will make sensible choices when deciding which simple carbs to ban from your diet entirely, which ones to limit your intake of, and which to enjoy on a weekly basis.

In Chapter 14: 'Sculpt your Body' we will speak about how exercise and lean muscle tissue can prevent too much glucose being stored as fat. The primary solution, however, is simply not to eat too much in the first place. The Pyramid sets limits for you to prevent this happening; so as long as you follow the pattern and adhere to Pyramid guidelines, you will not experience problems in this respect.

COMPLEX CARBOHYDRATES

Complex carbohydrates are the types of food often referred to as 'starchy foods'. As with simple carbs, they can exist in both natural and refined forms. For example, oats, wholegrains and chickpeas contain unrefined starches, whereas white bread, biscuits and pizza are refined starchy foods. By now you know it's the latter you need to avoid!

When it comes to bread, therefore, wholegrain is of course better than white, and granary and soya breads are the best options. There are also various brands of gluten- and sugar-free breads which present equal health benefits. Never buy bread containing added sugar, and save most bread for high-carb days.

As we've seen, all carbohydrates are digested to form glucose, whether they are simple or complex. When there is not enough glucose in your system, your body uses the hormone glucagon (also secreted by the pancreas) to convert any stored glycogen back into glucose. The more refined the carbohydrate, the faster the insulin trigger and the more peaks and troughs will occur in your blood-sugar levels.

Complex carbohydrates provide a slower and more sustained release of energy, making them better at suppressing your appetite and keeping you feeling full for longer. However, eating excessive quantities of any carbohydrates in one sitting will leave you feeling tired and lethargic, exactly the opposite of the intended effect. Sticking to Pyramid-sized portions of complex carbohydrates, and including fibrous carbs with your meal, will ensure you create the right balance for your body. This brings me on to the subject of vegetables, perhaps the single most important family of foods necessary for a healthy lifestyle.

FIBROUS CARBOHYDRATES

Most green vegetables are fibrous carbohydrates: they contain so much fibre and so little sugar or starch, that their carbohydrate content is more or less negated. As you'll learn in this section, the Pyramid Diet is based on net carbs, a figure which is reached by subtracting a food's fibre content from its total carb content. Fibrous vegetables are therefore not considered 'carbohydrates' for the purposes of calculating your daily carb intake.

Fibrous Vegetables

- Broccoli
- Spinach
- Leeks
- Green beans
- Cauliflower
- Courgette
- Spring onions
- Mushrooms

Starchy Vegetables

- Corn-on-the-cob
- Sweet potato
- Peas
- Yam
- Butter beans
- Chickpeas
- Kidney beans
- Lentils

As a general rule of thumb, the darker green the vegetables, the more fibre they contain. For example, spinach contains more fibre than lettuce, and broccoli more than celery. Why am I asking you to be consumed with this information? In a nutshell:

Fibre Helps You Lose Weight!

Fibre is a key component of any healthy diet. It works by pushing the food we eat through our systems because we are unable to break it down quickly in our stomachs. Once the food has passed through the digestive tract, we are able to eliminate waste effectively from our systems. Without fibre, undigested food stays in our stomachs too long and starts to release toxins into the body, causing stomach pains and even IBS. Ever wondered why you're suffering from a stomach-ache after that takeaway? Lack of fibre could well be the catalyst.

I suspect you're curious as to how eating *more* of something can help you to lose weight. There are various reasons for increasing our intake of fibre in our quest for slender perfection:

- Fibrous foods take longer to chew, reducing the amount of food you're likely to eat in one sitting.
- When the fibre reaches your stomach it acts like a sponge, soaking up water and creating a sense of fullness.
- Fibre takes longer to break down than most other foods, again producing satiating results. The impact this has on our appetites not only delays hunger, but also helps to conquer cravings.
- Most fibrous foods (especially vegetables) contain very few calories.
- Fibrous foods are normally low in fat, whilst being high in vitamins and minerals essential for an efficient metabolic system.

Most of us don't get enough fibre in our diets. Unsure whether you're eating enough? Take a look in your fridge and analyse the colours of the vegetables in front of you. The more colourful the selection, the more fibre you're likely to be getting. If you're short on time or perhaps travel too often to stock up on fresh vegetables, the good news is that, whilst canned and frozen alternatives will lose out on some nutrients, they do retain their dietary fibre. Just be sure to filter out any brands with added salt, sugar or other preservatives.

In previous chapters, we've spoken briefly about the terrible effect sugar can have on both our health and physical appearance, and the importance of a diet low in sugar-laden carbs. Choosing the wrong carbohydrates will counteract all of the positive effects the Pyramid Diet would otherwise have on your body.

Fruity Facts

A common topic of recent debate, and one that should be carefully considered when discussing 'the right carbs', is that of fruit consumption. Whilst some nutritionists still maintain that 'an apple a day keeps the doctor away', others have decided that the natural sugars in fruits mean they should be omitted from the shopping trolley entirely. Then there are those experts who attempt to guide us towards choosing certain fruits over others. With so many conflicting views and opinions flying around, it's not surprising many of us end up going bananas! Can Pyramid dieters eat fruit? Of course they can! So where has all this doubt stemmed from, and how much fruit should one consume in a day?

Fruit: Friend or Foe?

'A number of recent research studies recommend an increased intake of fruit to decrease the risk of obesity and related disorders. We are all familiar with the five-a-day campaign. However, an enormous amount of confusion has arisen amongst consumers, who are puzzled that fruit

MIGUEL SAYS ...

can apparently help manage their weight while also having a high sugar content.

'Most of the negative publicity surrounding fruit focuses on the specific type of sugar it contains, namely fructose. High-fructose corn syrups have been linked to the recent increase in obesity and obesity-related disorders. This contributes to energy production through aerobic metabolism, feeding into a complex set of reactions which produces adenosine triphosphate – ATP – the energy "currency" used by our cells. Under normal circumstances, any excess sugar – including fructose – is removed by the liver. However, when large amounts of sugar are eaten, the liver begins to produce lipids known as triglycerides, which in turn are deposited as fat.

'Please don't panic just yet about those two apples you ate this morning! Fructose from whole fruit is very different from that in corn syrups. Most fruit has a high water and fibre content, which means the fructose is diluted. Also, the fibre naturally found in whole fruits actually reduces the glycaemic load of that fruit, i.e. it slows the absorption of fructose into the bloodstream, so you're not getting a concentrated hit of fructose all at once.

'But the biggest benefit of the inclusion of fruit in the modern diet is its tendency to reduce a person's total daily intake. Fresh fruits possess many nutritional qualities which other high carbohydrate foods do not. They are low in calories, high in water content, and contain a large amount of dietary fibre, vitamins and minerals. When we consume fruit, the feeling of satiety occurs relatively early and lasts for a relatively long period of time. In addition, consuming a piece of fruit directly after a main meal will maximize the satiating effect of that meal, whilst minimizing its glycae-mic load. Low GL meals provide a sustained release of glucose into the bloodstream, again leading to prolonged satiety.

'For these reasons, consuming up to 4 portions of fresh fruit – especially directly after meals – has a truly positive impact on regulating your intake throughout the day. If you are a 'snacker' or 'grazer' and like fruit, I would advise you to combine it with a few nuts or a thin slice of low-fat cheese. By adding some protein to that snack you will maxi-mize its satiating effect, reducing your appetite for longer.'

So which fruits make the best addition to the Pyramid Diet? The GI content should be taken into consideration, as well as portion control when opting for grapes or berries. You will find fruity statistics listed in the tables in Chapter 16, but for now, here are some tips to get you started.

Low GI Fruits

Should you wish to take fruit in your bag to snack on at work or munch whilst on the go, there are a variety of juicy sweet options to choose from. In line with the rules of the Pyramid, I'd recommend apples, bananas, blueberries, black-berries, clementines, cranberries, pears, plums, strawberries and raspberries. One portion is either one piece of fruit, or one small handful of berries. Be careful when opting for bananas, as the calorie content of a large banana is two to three times that of an apple. Whilst you are not encouraged to be too calorie conscious on the Pyramid Diet, it does help to be informed of the composition of regular snacks.

High GI Fruits

There are some fruits best avoided due to their high GI value. These are dried figs, dates, currants and Cantaloupe melon. Make a mental note of this list, or take it with you to the supermarket in order to avoid 'innocent' mistakes when browsing the fruit and veg aisle! Swapping melon for berries may sound like an insignificant exchange, but the benefits of these simple tips all add up.

MIGUEL SAYS …

'Dried fruit contains more calories and natural sugars per helping because the dehydration process removes most of the water. That missing water means there are more pieces of dried fruit in the same serving. For example, 1 grape and 1 raisin both have 7 calories; however 1 *cup* of grapes has about 60 calories, while a cup of raisins has over 400.

'The sugar in dried fruit is fructose and glucose, the sugars that are naturally found in fresh fruit. But be sure to read labels before you buy – sometimes sugar is added to dried fruits like cranberries, since they're so tart. Obviously the extra sugar adds calories without any added nutritional value. You have to be careful with these so-called healthy snacks because you could be ingesting huge amounts of sugar. Furthermore, dried fruit has a higher GI than fresh fruit, and is often preserved using sulfites, which have allergenic properties.

'Look for bars that also include nuts because this combination will lower the glycaemic load of the snack.'

One final point to be made when it comes to fruit (and this is fundamental) is that because fruits are carbohydrate foods they are to be consumed on high- and low-carb days only, and definitely not on no-carb days. An average apple contains around 15g of net carbs, meaning you'd almost have hit your daily carb limit if you ate just one on a no-carb day. A banana has around 25g of net carbs; an even higher price to pay for one small snack. But remember, you can loosen your belt a little on the carb front on low-carb days, and even more so on high-carb days. Relax in the knowledge that once you become accustomed to the Pyramid method, you will subconsciously make selective food choices to suit certain days without even realizing you're doing it!

Sneaky Sugars

We've covered some of those sneaky hidden sugars, and now I'm going to give you enough detail to avoid them. Bearing in mind that ingredients are listed in order of weight, it's alarming to discover that numerous family favourites are full to the brim with sugar and additives. Not only that, these products are often promoted by the manufacturers as 'healthy options', and packaged in such a way as to lead us to believe they are probably sugar-free, or 'all natural'.

Remember the case of yoghurt vs doughnut from Chapter 2? The Krispy Kreme doughnut contained 16 fewer grams of sugar than the Yoplait yoghurt, which you'll recall is promoted as being '99% fat free'. This is not an isolated case. Peruse the health-food aisles of your local supermarket and you'll find that dozens of so-called 'healthier options' turn out to be full to the brim with added sugars.

Packaged foods containing any amount of added sugar simply don't have a place on the Pyramid Diet. The Food

Standards Agency (FSA) consider any product containing more than 15g of sugar per 100g to be 'high in sugar'. If in doubt, always refer back to the 'sugar alphabet' from Chapter 2 and remember to 'read before you feed'. In the meantime, here are some shockers to get your metabolic minds ticking.

Product	Advertising slogans and health claims	Sugar per 100g
Kellogg's Nutri-Grain Cereal Bar (apple and cinnamon)	'One good decision can lead to another.' 'Nutri-Grain. Eat better all day.'	32.4g
Kellogg's Special K Red Berries	'This cereal packs a few healthy vitamins into each and every morning.'	29g
Kellogg's All-Bran Bran Buds	'Made with natural wheat bran.' Provides '51% recommended daily fibre per serving.'	26.7g
Kellogg's Low Fat Granola With Raisins	'Low-fat multi-grain cereal.'	28.3g
Kellogg's Smart Start Strong Heart Toasted Oat cereal	'Good source of fibre. Made with whole grain.'	28.3g
Slim-Fast Chocolate Crunch Meal Bar	'Look good . . . feel great.' 'Eat six times a day and still lose weight.'	21g
Slim-Fast Chocolate Caramel Bar	'Look good . . . feel great.' 'Eat six times a day and still lose weight.'	48g
Slim-Fast Blissful Banana Flavour Powder	'Look good . . . feel great.' 'Eat six times a day and still lose weight.'	50g
Eat Natural Blueberry, Pistachio and Yoghurt Bar	'Packed with good, wholesome stuff . . . and nothing dodgy.'	38.2g
Eat Natural Breakfast Bar	'Packed with good, wholesome stuff . . . and nothing dodgy.'	24g
Nature Valley Oats and Hazelnuts Granola Bars	'Jam packed with wholegrain oats.'	23g
Nature Valley Oats 'n' Honey Granola Bars	'Jam packed with wholegrain oats.'	28.6g
South Beach Diet High Protein Cereal Bar (Chocolate)	'The Delicious, Doctor-Designed, Foolproof Weight-Loss Plan'	20g

These foods are all branded in a way which would have even the most diet-savvy among us believe they're good for our health. In reality, a cereal or bar embellished with images of fields, grass and trees is just as likely to give you a sugar overload as a blatantly naughty sweet treat. Natural sugars can be forgiven to an extent, but the items listed above are far from innocent.

In future, when purchasing packaged products, take heed of these words:

Green Does Not Mean Clean!

Stick instead to Pyramid-approved options such as plain old porridge oats, or brands like Quaker Oat So Simple Original (not the flavoured versions) or Jordans Chunky Traditional Porridge, adding cinnamon or fresh berries to taste. There are also a few Pyramid-approved snack bars available, although they should only be an occasional treat because, although they're natural, they are still high in sugar.

> 'Adding anything from ¼ to ½ a teaspoon of cinnamon to your porridge slows down the release of sugar into your bloodstream, effectively lowering the glycaemic load of that meal,' says Miguel Toribio-Mateas.

MIGUEL SAYS ...

4. Protein Perfection

I've already outlined the importance of protein in the Pyramid Diet and you'll recall that you should aim to consume at least 1g per lb of body weight per day. But when it comes to choosing the best forms of protein, there is still some groundwork to be done.

You may have come across low-carb diets that allow for the consumption of burgers and sausages from any old meat factory, but for both nutritional and ethical reasons, the Pyramid Diet is not one of them. Please don't be tempted to skim-read this section or ignore this advice! Read on, then make your own decisions, but I hope you'll appreciate the significance of what follows.

Is Beef Black and White?

In short, no. We as humans may be at the top of the food chain, but we are still a link. Consequently we are also a party to the diet of the cow (or whichever animal we happen to consume), and not all beef minces up the same way in our bodies. This first came to my attention when reading an article about top body-builder John Meadows, founder of the Mountain Dog Diet.* After experimenting on his own body, John reported: 'The first thing I did was swap regular

* 'To burn fat: the Mountain Dog diet helps you accomplish generally disparate

beef for grass-fed beef, and my waist got smaller. I had some other people try it, and I measured their waists – they all got smaller.'

Although the reasons for this are not entirely clear, John suspected it may have been because grass-fed beef has 3 to 5 times higher levels of CLA (conjugated linoleic acid), a fat-burning chemical that may also reduce the risk of developing certain cancers.* Not only that, grass-fed beef is richer in omega-3 and lower in omega-6 than grain-fed beef, a benefit for most Westerners, who tend to lack the former and ingest too much of the latter. Free-range and organic meat is also leaner, not only because the animals are fed a healthy diet, but because they get much more exercise than caged animals.

Just to be clear, when I use the term 'leaner', there is more significance than merely saving you cutting off the odd piece of fat. A 6oz steak from a grass-fed cow can have 100 fewer calories than a 6oz steak from a grain-fed cow. It is typical for meat-lovers to consume around 66½lbs of beef per year, or just over 177 of those steaks. This means that switching to lean grass-fed beef will save you about 17,700 calories a year without the need for any dietary willpower or deprivation. Taking this into account, even if everything else in your diet stayed exactly the same, you'd shed approximately 6lbs per

---

goals – looking like a bodybuilder and getting healthy' by Sean Hyson, *Muscle & Fitness*, July 2011.

* A Finnish study in 2000 found older women with the highest levels of CLA in their diets had a 60 per cent lower risk of developing breast cancer than women with the lowest CLA. ('Inverse association between dietary and serum conjugated linoleic acid and risk of breast cancer in postmenopausal women,' Aro, Mannisto *et al.*, *Nutrition and Cancer*, vol. 38, 2000)

year by making the switch. If that's not weight-loss handed to you on a plate then I don't know what is!

Yes, grass-fed meat does come with a higher price tag than standard meat, but in my view it is well worth it. It is very difficult to source 100 per cent grass-fed beef in mainstream supermarkets, but my research into what is available is reassuring and means that even if you're on a fairly tight budget or have a large family to feed, eating free-range or organic meat can still be done. Whilst these cattle have not been reared entirely on grass, their diets come a lot closer to the ideal than standard meat. For example, Tesco's 'Finest' beef comes from cows which are reared on grass for a minimum of six months alongside their mothers, and I personally believe this is 'good enough' in the quest for grass-fed proteins. However, if you wish to buy meat from animals fed solely on grass, there are a number of high-quality online stores which deliver to your door.

Minced meat is an economic option which is also very versatile. At the time of going to press, 500g of free-range minced beef costs less than £3, and would typically make four delicious quarter-pounder beefburgers, or a wholewheat spaghetti bolognese large enough for the entire family. Beef mince is also great for making meatballs or chilli con carne. When you add the cost of any accompanying ingredients, these dishes come in at less than £2 a head. Turn to the recipe pages in Chapter 15 if you fancy giving any of these quick and easy recipes a go.

So where beef is concerned: never buy cheap meat or burgers from fast-food chains, buy grass-fed wherever possible, and always opt for lean cuts.

The Chicken and the Egg

Selecting the right chicken can also be a complex task if you don't know what to look out for. But does our choice of chicken really affect our waistlines?

Just like any other animal, when chickens are housed indoors and deprived of greens, their meat becomes low in precious omega-3s, as do their eggs. This is the first good reason to buy free-range or organic produce and steer clear of caged hens. The second (and this applies to all meat) is the fact that there is far more CLA in free-range pasture-fed meat than caged meat.

Flavoured 'ready to cook' chickens are very rarely free-range. They may look tempting and seem cheap, but the price always reflects the quality of the product. The same can often be said for imported meat. Don't give in to chicken burgers from fast-food chains, or cheap imported meats, even if they do claim to be made from 100 per cent chicken breast. These products are often pumped full of water to increase the weight and have chemicals added for preservation and taste purposes.

When the BBC investigated this in 2003, the findings were shocking. About 40 per cent of the imported chicken sold by catering suppliers undergoes heavy processing. Whilst this meat appears fresh and plump, it is rubbery and tasteless, known in the trade as 'plastic chicken'. The majority of this meat comes from Holland and Belgium and can be enhanced with water, chemicals and even pig's skin. Much of it is distributed to takeaway restaurants, so before ordering always be sure to ask the waiter if they use British meat.

Lesson learned? When it comes to chicken, eat fresh, eat free-range and eat British!

Save Your Bacon

Whether it's bacon and eggs, sausage sandwiches or a traditional pork roast, it all begins with a pig. There has been a lot of speculation in recent years surrounding the welfare of these animals, and rightly so. Many of you will have seen the 2009 TV series *Jamie Saves Our Bacon*, in which Jamie Oliver investigated the gruesome truth behind imported pork, the chemicals that go into the products and the unthinkable conditions the animals are kept in. Thankfully, action has been taken to ensure we now know exactly what we're buying.

In October 2011 a £2 million national marketing campaign was launched, with slogans such as 'Grill It Before you Buy It' and 'No More Porkies', to encourage consumers to look for the Red Tractor mark, which guarantees that high standards are met when it comes to the animals' feed, their slaughter and the production of sausages, bacon, gammon and ham. The logo covers not only pork, but other meats and food products too.

Whilst British farmers do us proud and operate some of the highest animal-welfare standards in the world, this is sadly not the case in many other countries. Supermarkets continue to stock imported meat from countries operating far lower standards, which in turn have cheaper production costs. An estimated two-thirds of imported pork and pork products are produced in a way that would be illegal in Britain. That's more than enough gruesome information to encourage me to buy British, and I hope it sways you too.

Aside from the welfare of the pigs we eat, there are also many health benefits in keeping cheap pork away from our plates. Pork often receives more flak than it deserves. Many people favour chicken from a health point of view, but in fact, whilst chicken contains slightly more protein, good-quality, lean cuts of pork come very close and the B vitamins they contain play a vital role in the functioning of our metabolisms, helping to keep excess weight at bay. Pork tenderloin, pork fillet and lean pork chops are the most healthy choices; minced or diced pork tends to be quite fatty and of poor quality. As with beef and chicken, free-range or organic pork will provide you with greater nutritional benefits than 'value' or imported products. When it comes to meat, you definitely do get what you pay for!

So how about sausages and bacon? Do they have a place on the Pyramid Diet? Of course they do, you just need to be very selective when it comes to these products. Cheap sausages and fatty rashers of bacon worm their way into supermarkets, work canteens, builders' cafés and fast-food restaurants the world over. Just one bite and we seem to be hooked. But consider the truth behind these products, and I hope you will never touch this grease again.

In the UK, the minimum meat content required for a product to be labelled 'pork sausages' is 42 per cent, although that 'pork' can itself contain 30 per cent fat and 25 per cent connective tissue. Where meat content does not meet this minimum requirement, the product is simply labelled 'sausages'. It is imperative you are aware of this, because these 'sausages' can be made up of skin, gristle, bone and MRM (mechanically recovered meat), obtained by removing residual meat from bones using a high-pressure machine. One word: yuk! The most common use of MRM is in hot dogs, which

I urge you to steer clear of altogether. Your body will thank you for not stuffing it full of fatty, gristly pieces of poor-quality meat which have been pumped full of chemicals. Never has there been a better reason to read before you feed!

Lamb: Should We Give it the Chop?

Lamb has a reputation for being fatty, and many critics advise us to axe it in favour of leaner sources of protein, claiming it has no place on the healthy British menu. However, lambs are generally not subjected to overcrowded, inhumane conditions, nor are they pumped full of chemicals. In this respect, it may be the safest bet of all the meats we've touched on so far.

All red meat, including lamb, is an excellent source of alpha lipoic acid (ALA), a nutrient also found in foods such as broccoli and spinach, and a powerful antioxidant. It is essential for good health, helping us to burn glucose by converting it to energy. If your body were lacking ALA supplies, you'd be unable to muster any energy at all. Sufficient stores of ALA, on the other hand, cause a decrease in glucose and insulin levels, reducing insulin resistance and in turn lowering your risk of developing diabetes. Think about it; the more glucose we burn, the less insulin we secrete and therefore the less fat our bodies will be inclined to store.

There are many other nutritional benefits to eating lamb. A 3oz portion provides 30 per cent of the RDA of zinc, essential for growth, healing and a healthy immune system. It is also a good source of iron, which is vital for the formation of red blood cells. Both iron and zinc are more easily absorbed from red meat than other sources. Lamb is also a great source of B vitamins, essential for metabolic reactions – and by now you don't need me to tell you what this means when it comes to unwanted weight! Finally, today's lamb is much leaner than it was twenty years ago. Thanks to modern farming and production methods, so long as you buy lean cuts and remove the fat you can see, the lamb that lands on your plate is likely to be lean enough to pass the Pyramid test.

Despite the benefits associated with lamb, there are many other meats which can offer a more favourable protein–fat ratio. Read on to find out which ones come top of the Pyramid.

A Walk on the Wild Side

We've covered the most popular meats in the British kitchen, but it's well worth thinking outside the box. Meats such as venison and rabbit have an awful lot to offer, not only in terms of flavour, but crucially in fighting the flab. Take a look at the table below to see the variety of healthy and nutritious cuts.*

Meat	Protein per 100g	Fat per 100g	Carbs per 100g	Calories per 100g	Pyramid star-rating
Beef (lean)	22.7g	2g	0g	152	****
Lamb (lean)	20.8g	5.7g	0g	167	**
Pork (lean)	22.3g	4.9g	0g	165	**

* Figures taken from www.juxtable.com

Meat	Protein per 100g	Fat per 100g	Carbs per 100g	Calories per 100g	Pyramid star-rating
Chicken	24.4g	1.9g	0g	121	****
Venison (wild)	23.7g	1.4g	0g	149	****
Duck (wild)	19.9g	4.3g	0g	180	**
Rabbit (wild)	21.8g	2.4g	0g	144	***
Turkey	25.7g	1.1g	0g	163	*****
Pheasant (wild)	25.7g	0.6g	0g	148	*****

The Pyramid Diet is not only about losing weight and keeping it off, it is also about introducing you to new foods. If you normally play it safe in the meat department, I urge you to try turkey and wild game, which present an array of health benefits.

TURKEY

Traditionally a Christmas meat, turkey barely gets a look-in for eleven months of the year. This is a great shame when it contains more protein and less fat than chicken. It is also cheaper to buy. So next time you're doing the weekly shop, why not give turkey a try?

WILD GAME

Wild game such as venison and pheasant packs a pretty impressive profile, topping the chart for both highest protein content and lowest fat content per serving. Whilst unfortunately it is not widely available in the supermarket, there are plenty of specialist stores that stock game. If game is not something you've tried before, turn to Chapter 15 for some delicious and simple recipe ideas.

Plenty of Fish in the Sea

We have so many species of seafood to choose from, but often shy away from purchasing those we are unfamiliar with, or that require preparation before cooking. Don't be afraid to try new things, because when it comes to seafood you could be missing out on something you really enjoy. I believe there's a type of fish for everyone. And I'm not talking about battered cod from the local fish and chip shop!

Oily fish such as salmon, mackerel and sardines are the best sources of omega-3 because it's in a form that can be used by our bodies immediately. Oily fish also offer an excellent source of protein. If you're still unsure, look at the recipes in Chapter 15, where you're bound to find something that tickles your taste buds.

I accept that some people don't get on with oily fish. If you're one of them, bear in mind that white fish tend to have a milder taste and a less 'fishy' aroma. To help you find the fish that's right for you, I urge you to try some recipes from this book. The protein contents of the most popular seafoods are in the tables in Chapter 16.

'There is no doubt that animal proteins have a superior amino-acid profile to that of vegetarian sources. However, if you don't want to eat meat that often and you're not keen on cottage cheese, it is absolutely fine to eat fish every day – the Japanese have been doing it for centuries!

'Fish and seafood are also amongst the best sources of

MIGUEL SAYS ...

iodine, an essential mineral for the production of thyroxine, which regulates your metabolism. Subclinical hypothyroid, i.e. less-than-ideal function that doesn't require medical treatment as yet, is one of the conditions I most frequently see in my clinic. Most people presenting hypothyroid symptoms are overweight, and the introduction of larger amounts of fish and seafoods into their diets has a massive beneficial impact. Choose from a variety of different sea-food and alternate white and oily fish to bring a good range of proteins into your daily diet, whilst supporting the health of your thyroid,' says Miguel Toribio-Mateas.

The Nuts and Bolts

You'll find lots of alternative sources of protein in Chapter 10, 'The Pyramid for Vegetarians and Vegans', but below are a few further suggestions to help you boost your protein power throughout the day:

- Nuts
- Cottage cheese
- Low-fat yoghurt
- Roasted chickpeas
- Low-fat cheese
- Protein shakes
- Hummus
- Peanut, cashew or almond butter

5. Dairy, Fats and Drinks

Milk: A Cloudy Debate

I've no doubt that most of you are a little uncertain whether or not to include milk in your diet. Popular coffee chains present us with so many options when it comes to our morning brew. 'Skinny', 'soya' and 'light' are all terms which regularly crop up on their menus. But which one are we supposed to choose when watching our weight? Or should we cut out milk altogether in favour of a simple black coffee or herbal tea?

On to the facts. Would it surprise you to learn that milk contains sugar? I'm sorry to drop a bombshell, but if you thought you'd eradicated sugar from your diet by ditching refined carbs and avoiding the office vending machine, you're probably not quite there yet! Milk contains its own natural form of sugar called lactose. Not only does this have to be taken into consideration when calculating your carbohydrate consumption, intolerance to lactose is extremely common.

'If you have fair skin and blue, green or grey eyes and are of European descent, you are most likely to have lactase persistance, a genetic polymorphism or variation that makes you less able to digest milk and milk products. The positive trade-off from this evolutionary adaptation is that you're more able to absorb Vitamin D from the sun, so look on the bright side!'

MIGUEL SAYS …

Most of us who suffer from a lactose-induced irritation are totally oblivious to the condition, although it can lead to all manner of uncomfortable symptoms, such as bloating, cramps, diarrhoea, flatulence and nausea. The problem arises because of the body's inability to produce enough of the enzyme lactase, which helps it to absorb the milk. If you think you may be unable to properly digest lactose, strike milk off your shopping list without a second thought. If your suspicions were correct, you'll soon notice those ghastly symptoms you were experiencing have disappeared.

Just think about it; the only time we need milk is when we are babies. The same goes for cows, goats and sheep. Have you ever witnessed a grown cow drinking milk from a bucket? Of course not! The calf, kid or lamb suckles its mother's teat until it grows old enough to eat solid food, such as grass. At this time, the animal will progress to drinking only water, the only fluid essential for life. We as humans are no more than animals and subsequently we function in exactly the same way. Drinking cow's, goat's and sheep's milk as adults may be something we've done for centuries, but that doesn't mean to say it's good for us. It is certainly not what nature intended, which goes some way towards explaining such widespread intolerance to lactose.

If you do 'get on' with cow's milk, opt for skimmed milk on account of its relatively low calorific value. If you think you might be intolerant, you can now get milk which has had the lactase enzyme added ('Lactofree', available from Waitrose and others). If you decide to exclude milk from your diet altogether, try unsweetened soya milk, which is a godsend for those of us who are lactose intolerant but enjoy white tea and coffee. Soya (or soy) milk is made from soy beans and contains only vegetable proteins. Not only does it taste delicious, the vegetable protein it contains has been shown to decrease cholesterol levels. Even more significantly, it contains isoflavones, which help prevent osteoporosis, reduce the risk for certain cancers and ease menopausal symptoms.

If soya is just not to your taste, a good compromise is goat's milk because the fat particles contained in it are smaller than those in cow's milk, making it easier to digest and the vitamins and minerals easier to absorb.

Dairy Products

You don't need me to tell you that if you are lactose intolerant it's not advisable to eat products made with milk. But for the dairy devils amongst you who are able to consume milk-based products, which ones will put the brakes on fat loss, and which ones are welcome additions to your diet?

CHEESE

Cheddar, Edam, Stilton and Brie are just a small selection of the most popular cheeses found in UK supermarkets, restaurants and delicatessens. Most of us like cheese and eat it in one form or another, be it as an ingredient in a rich dessert such as cheesecake, as a lunchbox snack, in a sandwich or burger, or as part of an extravagant cheeseboard. But does cheese make you fat?

Well, it's pretty simple! A 100g serving of cheddar cheese packs a whopping 34g of fat and over 400 calories. So full-fat cheddar is out, but there are a number of low-fat options available for cheese-lovers. Just make sure when selecting low-fat cheese that it really is marked 'low', in line with FSA guidelines; the calorie content will come down accordingly.

A much better choice is cottage cheese, popular among the body-building community because it's high in protein and reasonably low in fat: a 100g serving contains around 13g of protein and 4g of fat. Cottage cheese is also very versatile, and makes a great addition to green salads, fruity snacks, meat-based recipes and desserts. The net-carb content of cottage cheese is very low, so provided you're careful, there's no reason you can't enjoy it on any of the three days.

MIGUEL SAYS …

'When looking at different sources of protein, it can be helpful to consider their biological value (BV), a value between 0 and 100 which is determined by their amino-acid composition, an indicator of how easily your body can digest the protein and use it to build other proteins. Cottage cheese is known as a "complete protein" with a very high BV (85–90), which means that it contains all of the amino acids that your body requires to build muscle. Muscle is the tissue that burns the most calories, so cottage cheese is an excellent choice for those of you wanting to increase muscle mass and stay lean.'

YOGHURT

This is a tricky one. Yoghurt can do wonders for your body, but can also be a dietary disaster if you allow yourself to fall foul of sales jargon. There are so many yoghurts on the market aimed specifically at those of us who watch our weight, that we find ourselves dodging a minefield of manufacturers' claims, forever wondering which brand will truly help us beat the bulge. I've said it before and I'll say it again: '99 per cent fat free' does not mean sugar-free and therefore does not mean the product is good for your health. There are dozens of so-called 'healthy' yoghurts on the market just waiting to jump off the chiller cabinet and into our shopping bags. As a rule of thumb, it's the fat-free yoghurts you need to be wary of, as these often contain more sugar than traditional yoghurt. Just remember: *read before you feed*! Refer back to the sugar alphabet in Chapter 2 if you're unsure whether a specific ingredient listed on the pot is indeed a type of sugar.

Eating the right yoghurt does have benefits. Plain yoghurt, or yoghurt with no added sugar makes a great snack or dessert on a high-carb day. Remember to check the label to be sure it has no artificial flavourings or additives. The best yoghurts are those containing live bacteria, which offer a whole host of health benefits. To begin with, the lactose is converted by the bacteria into lactic acid, which helps your body digest it and may mean you can eat it without experiencing discomfort. Not only this, the calcium in yoghurt can be absorbed by the body much more effectively than other milk products, because calcium needs to enter the body in an acid matrix. As you've just learned, yoghurt converts lactose into lactic acid, making it the perfect candidate to maximize calcium absorption.

The advantages of eating yoghurt do not end there. It is rich in potassium, protein and B vitamins, including B12. It can also help strengthen and stabilize the immune system, provided you choose a brand offering 'live cultures'. There are plenty of low-fat plain yoghurts available in all major supermarkets, health-food stores and online.

'Live cultures in yoghurt are naturally probiotic. They help optimize bowel health and support immune function. Goat's and sheep's yoghurt tend to have a more interesting culture mix which contribute to a happier, flatter stomach.'*

So yoghurt containing live bacteria can be consumed in moderation on any given day. The carbohydrate content is reduced, because the live bacteria helps lower the carb load you'd otherwise be consuming from the lactose. Fruit-flavoured yoghurts have a higher carb content, though, and are more likely to have sugar added, so if you crave a hint of fruitiness, just add fresh fruit yourself on high-carb days.

CREAM AND ICE CREAM

As you probably suspected, cream and ice cream are not on the menu. But I do have some good news for you, in the form of tasty Pyramid-approved alternatives that can be found in the tables in Chapter 16.

BUTTER, SPREADS AND OILS

Nowadays we are inundated with advertisements for spreads, all claiming to be more healthy than traditional butter and oils. There are so many products to choose from, and too

---

* There is currently no scientific consensus on these claims. E.g., see the Wiki entries for Probiotics, Actimel and Yakult for an overview plus relevant studies.

many other aspects of our health to concern ourselves with to find time to enter into margarine wars. For this reason, I suggest we make sound, simple decisions and stick with them.

When you need to use oil for dressings or cold dishes, always opt for extra-virgin olive oil. It may be more expensive than some more popular brands of oils and spreads, but the little changes go a long way towards losing weight and keeping it off. If you can't shake the urge for a spread on your bread, try lightly drizzling the extra-virgin olive oil then spreading with a knife, and embrace the Mediterranean flavours.

Olive oil can be damaged when heated and its health benefits negated, so if you're cooking you should use an oil which is able to withstand high heats, such as safflower or sunflower oil. In my opinion, though, the very best is the extra-virgin olive oil spray produced by FryLight, which has Vitamin E added to prevent oxidation when cooking, so it is safe to use at high temperatures.

Fight Fat With Fat

As a Pyramid follower, you are encouraged to include a healthy amount of good fats in your daily diet. Low-fat diets, as previously discussed, are not conducive to healthy and sustainable weight-loss. As we've seen, all too often 'low fat' or '99 per cent fat free' foods contain stacks of added sugar, which is in fact more detrimental to weight-loss than fat itself.

On the Pyramid Diet we learn to fight fat with fat. 'Cutting down on fat too much can cause vitamin deficiency,' says Miguel Toribio-Mateas. 'Fat-soluble vitamins like A, E, K and COQ10 are essential for energy and for beautiful skin. This is what low-fat diets fail to recognize.'

So which fats are 'good fats' and which types should you cut down on? I've mentioned omega-3 and omega-6 already, but now I'll explain exactly why these are such indispensable fats.

PUFAs

Omega-3 and omega-6 are polyunsaturated fatty acids (PUFAs), essential fatty acids which cannot be made by the body and so must be consumed in our diets. Both are capable of being metabolized to form long-chain PUFAs.

OMEGA-3

Numerous studies have shown omega-3 long-chain PUFAs help maintain a healthy heart and cardiovascular system. They are also beneficial to bones, joints and the brain. Omega-3 fats help transfer oxygen around the body, relax blood vessels, reduce inflammation and even speed up the wound-healing process. They are also vital for healthy eyes, gut function, hormone production and, you guessed it, weight-loss! It is these properties which make omega-3 a well-deserved essential fatty acid, yet most of us do not get enough of it. Whilst there is no official RDA (recommended daily allowance) for omega-3, I'd strongly suggest you try to consume it from either plant or fish sources daily.

You already know that the best, complex form of omega-3 is found in oily fish and consists of two types of acids: EPA (eicosapentaenoic acid) and DHA (docosahexaenoic acid). Omega-3 is also present in plant sources such as nuts and seeds, but must then be converted into EPA and DHA. Foods such as eggs, grass-fed meats (such as beef from grazing cattle), flaxseed oil, walnuts and pumpkin seeds all offer respectable sources of omega-3. Another good source is the New Zealand green-lipped mussel.

Pyramid followers are encouraged to get plenty of this essential fat and there are various ways to do this. However, I often come across an adversity to cooking, preparing and even tasting oily fish. Mackerel and sardines do have a very distinctive taste, and if you don't like them, I can't force you to! If you do like them, then great – most supermarkets and of course fishmongers sell mackerel and sardine fillets to save you the messy and time-consuming job of preparing them at home. And if you're short on time or looking for something you can take to work with you, why not grab a tin or pouch of salmon? Tuna is also an option, but is not as rich in omega-3.

For those of you who truly can't face eating fish, select your favourite sources of omega-3 from the list above and ensure that it is one of your daily priorities. Another excellent alternative is krill oil, which provides an even better source of omega-3 and additional antioxidants to help ward off free radicals. Krill are shrimp-like crustaceans between 1 and 6cm long. In Japan, they are a popular food choice, and the oil extracted from them is becoming an increasingly popular nutritional supplement worldwide. It is widely available in capsule form in most good health-food stores and online.

OMEGA-6

Omega-6 fatty acids have the opposite effect on the body to omega-3. Whilst hormones derived from omega-3 decrease inflammation, blood clotting and cell proliferation, hormones from omega-6 actually increase these functions.

'Every cell in our body is surrounded by a cell membrane composed mainly of fatty acids. Cell membranes allow proper amounts of vital nutrients to enter the cell, whilst allowing waste products to be removed. Glucose is cleared from the bloodstream by insulin. It enters cells via specific receptors in the cell membrane. Omega-6 is responsible for cell membrane rigidity, and omega-3 for its fluidity. The ideal omega-6 to omega-3 ratio in our diet is 4:1. This ratio guarantees optimal fatty acid balance and minimizes the risk of developing insulin resistance, where your cells stop responding to insulin, allowing sugars to circulate in the bloodstream, in turn allowing more triglycerides (fat) to be released by the liver, and ultimately creating more fat around our middles. So an optimal fatty-acid ratio is paramount to avoid piling up the pounds!'

Although it is important for human health and something that must be present in our diets, in the Western world we actually consume too much omega-6 in relation to omega-3. As Miguel says above, the optimum ratio is 4:1; yet in the UK, the ratio is nearer 8:1. So most of us will need to concentrate on increasing our omega-3 consumption. Even so, we'll briefly touch on the best sources of omega-6.

Omega-6 fatty acids are found in seeds and nuts, and the oils extracted from them. Walnuts, brazil nuts, pecans, almonds, pumpkin, sunflower and sesame seeds are all good sources. If you're wondering how we can possibly be ingesting plenty of omega-6, it's because these things are often included in poor-quality food items such as cakes, breads and biscuits. Unfortunately, as a rule these are also full of salt, sugar and refined flours which are not favourable when following any kind of healthy eating plan and most definitely do not come with a Pyramid-approved stamp!

OMEGA-9

There is one more group of essential fatty acids, omega-9 (mono-unsaturated fatty acids). Unlike omega-3 and omega-6, they are produced by the body without the need for dietary supplementation.

Omega-9 has been proved to increase our levels of good cholesterol (HDL) and decrease our levels of bad cholesterol (LDL). This in turn helps to prevent or eliminate a build-up of plaque in the arteries. Plaque build-up can lead to heart attacks and strokes, so omega-9 is really quite significant to our health. Omega-9 fatty acids are found in vegetable and animal fats, most commonly in canola oil, olive oil, almonds and sunflower oil.

'All cooking oils are a mix of polyunsaturated and mono-unsaturated fatty acids. They have delicate chemical structures which are easily damaged by light and heat. This can turn a really healthy oil into a nasty pro-oxidant substance. Use little or no oil for cooking, or use a healthy vegetable oil like FryLight olive-oil spray, or any made from raw coconut. To get the full benefits from olive oil, use it raw by drizzling it on salads or on your cooked food. Another great salad oil with the perfect 4:1 ratio of omega-6 to omega-3 is hemp oil.'

MIGUEL SAYS ...

Hopefully you now feel clued-up on the importance of friendly fats and understand the reasons for including a healthy dose of these in your daily diet. Fat is notorious in the modern world for being responsible for high cholesterol and heart disease, yet cutting good fats out of your diet means you will have no protection from the same. So, protect your heart with Pyramid-approved sources of omega-3 and elevate oily fish and krill oil to the top of your priority list.

SFAs (Saturated Fatty Acids)

These are generally found in foods which remain solid at room temperature, such as butter, cream and cheese. Fatty animal meats and treats such as chocolate also tend to have a high saturated-fat content. The FSA (Food Standards Agency) warns that most of us eat about 20 per cent more than the recommended maximum amount of saturated fat. This can lead to high cholesterol, which in turn increases the risk of heart disease. For guidance, an item of food containing more than 5g saturates per 100g is considered by the FSA to be high in saturated fat. It goes without saying you should steer well clear of these foods, regardless of whether or not they are low in carbs. Foods containing 1.5g saturates or less per 100g are considered low in saturated fat. These are the foods you should opt for. Anything in between these two figures contains a medium amount of saturated fat. These foods are permissible in moderation on low- and no-carb days.

Once you become a Pyramid follower, you will quickly learn to make the right choices when it comes to dietary fats. Refined carbohydrates are often high in saturated fats too and are your biggest enemy. The combination of processed sugars and SFAs is lethal over a lifetime. In my opinion, these foods should be locked away behind the counter with cigarettes! Unfortunately, the reality is quite the opposite. Supermarkets tend to place these products in the most attractive locations, on offer at the end of aisles and beautifully stacked together as school lunchbox options. It's no wonder many parents are oblivious to the damage these foods can do to their children. The supermarkets do now colour-code food labels to help the consumer understand the nutritional content, but it's up to you to make sense of the overall package.

Thankfully, the Pyramid Diet generally banishes most packaged items to the bin, so a refined carb and SFA combination should not find its way into your trolley.

Sauces and Condiments

When you need a little flavour or spice in your life, it's time to get saucy. Some dishes are simply too dry or bland to be eaten without condiments. If we had the luxury of time to make these sauces from scratch, that would be ideal, but of course most of us use ready-made, and below is a quick assessment of the sauces we use most frequently. Can't find what you're looking for? If it's Pyramid-approved, chances are you'll find it in the tables in Chapter 16.

TOMATO KETCHUP

Ketchup is harmless as a concept: a spoonful of puréed tomatoes on the plate hardly equates to killer calories. However, you need to be wary of the popular brands as they contain a lot of added sugar and salt. If you're craving ketchup, opt for a reduced salt and sugar-free version.

VINEGAR

Vinegar makes a fabulous addition to a host of healthy recipes, some of which feature in Chapter 15. But there are so many different types of vinegar, which one should you choose? In my view, the best option is brown-rice vinegar. Rice vinegar offers more health benefits than standard commercial vinegars and contains twenty amino acids, thought to help destroy free radicals, which would otherwise contribute to premature aging, cancer and other degenerative diseases. Furthermore, brown-rice vinegar can also reduce cravings for sweet foods and suppress appetite, particularly if consumed before meals.*

MUSTARD

Most mustards are perfectly fine to have in moderation. I'd recommend Dijon mustard for its full flavour, and wholegrain mustard, with its wonderful grainy texture.

PICKLE

Some pickles are OK, but steer clear of the sweet varieties, which are high in sugar and carbs. If in doubt, read before you feed.

MAYONNAISE

Mayonnaise is heavy on calories and normally contains added salt and sugar. If you want to make your own with extra-

* 'Is Vinegar An Appetite Suppressant?' David L. Katz, MD, O, *The Oprah Magazine*, January 2007.

virgin olive oil, this is an option, but I'm afraid most shop-bought mayonnaises are simply empty calories. The same can be said for most other white sauces, such as salad cream.

BROWN SAUCE

Brown sauce is to be avoided. It tastes sugary and artificial because it is sugary and artificial. Strike this one off your list!

APPLE, CRANBERRY AND REDCURRANT SAUCES

Again, these sauces need to be home-made to avoid unnecessarily high sugar content.

HONEY AND JAM

Honey is a tricky one because the sugars it contains are natural, leading us to believe it's probably OK to eat. However, with an incredible 80g of sugar per 100g, I hope you'll soon change your mind. Honey is a real Pyramid no-no!

Jam is also *very* sugary and best left on the shelf for someone else.

NUT BUTTERS

Cashew, almond and peanut butters all make for delicious high-protein spreads, or additions to sauces. When choosing your brand, be sure it contains no added sugar. Always go easy on these products as they are extremely high in fat.

SOY SAUCE

Rich in vitamin B3 and amino acids, soy sauce is a great condiment to use in the Pyramid Diet. There are many different types, but 'tamari' is a dark, rich Japanese soy sauce which contains little or no wheat, making it ideal for those who are wheat-intolerant or seeking to reduce bloating. You also need to be aware of the high salt-content of soy sauce. Opt for reduced-salt brands where possible.

Can Drinks Make a Difference?

Hot Drinks: A Comfort or a Curse?

Can't live without your morning cuppa? Or perhaps you fail to function if you're deprived of your coffee kick? Tea and coffee are certainly addictive, but with the never-ending speculation surrounding the impact these drinks have on our health, should we continue to enjoy them, or would it be wiser to cut them out of our lives for good?

Should you wish to skip the science, I'd advise you to take tea over coffee, but both are OK in moderation. Without complicating matters unnecessarily, I've created a quick profile of both:

TEA

Pros

- Moderate caffeine intake is associated with the regulation of body-weight.

- Both black and green tea reduce glucose levels.
- Green tea has cholesterol-lowering properties.

Cons

- The side-effects associated with drinking tea only exist in extreme cases when it is consumed in vast quantities. Up to four cups of tea with skimmed milk per day is highly unlikely to do any long-term damage to your health, or cause weight-gain.

COFFEE

Pros

- Moderate caffeine intake is associated with the regulation of body-weight.
- Coffee contains antioxidants.
- Coffee can enhance fat-burning, especially when consumed pre-workout.

Cons

- Coffee raises glucose levels.
- Coffee can increase cortisol levels, which in turn can lead to weight-gain, particularly around the midriff.

If you're willing to make a positive change on this front, green tea is an excellent substitute because of its antioxidant properties. Fancy hot drinks from coffee shops are an absolute no-no. The amount of milk, syrup, cream and sugar in these concoctions is ghastly. Stick to tea (green, black or herbal) and coffee, and if you wish to take milk, use skimmed.

The odd soya or 'skinny' latte is acceptable on rare occasions, but otherwise the sugar and calories we ingest from these drinks are simply not worth it.

If you really cannot bear unsweetened tea or coffee, use xylitol as an alternative to table sugar or the more common sweeteners, which are also prohibited for their own reasons.

MIGUEL SAYS …

> 'Minimize the glycaemic impact of your coffee or tea by having that drink at the end of a main meal. If you choose to have a caffeine drink with a snack, make sure that you include a source of protein, e.g. nuts. You are less likely to disturb your blood-sugar levels this way.'

Fruit Juice: An Easy Way to Get Your Five-a-Day?

Fruit juice and fruit smoothies are very popular soft drinks, often presumed to be a healthy alternative to fizzy drinks. The government initiative to encourage us to eat 'five a day' has given the juice industry an enormous boost, as many manufacturers are able to say their product provides us with one of our five-a-day. Drinking a glass of fruit juice is also much more convenient than munching on an apple or steaming fresh vegetables. However, all that juice could be doing you more harm than good.

> 'Any processing of fruit, including juicing, increases its GI and GL, and therefore its impact on blood-sugar levels. Juicing strips away valuable fibre from the fruit pulp which reduces satiety. This means that having a whole piece of

fruit will delay the return of your appetite for longer than a glass of fruit juice. This seems to be particularly true of oranges, where research has shown a significantly smaller insulin response to whole fruit than to juice. The insulin and sugar responses to fruit depend on the fibre content; the more fibre, the more sustained the sugar release, which not only keeps the weight off, but translates into sustained energy levels, a vital point for those of you who suffer from fluctuating energy levels throughout the day. Most people are better off avoiding fruit juice.'

Fizzy Drinks

Low-cal or no-cal fizzy drinks are controversial. They contain almost no calories and use sweeteners instead of sugar, so how can they possibly contribute to weight-gain? The *Daily Express* newspaper recently splashed a feature entitled 'DIET DRINKS MAKE YOU FAT'. This article was the subject of much speculation, with many people (including some health experts) rubbishing the claims. However, there are a couple of reasons why diet drinks could be having an impact on our weight.

Firstly, the sweetener in diet drinks is thought to trigger the release of insulin in just the same way as sugar because our bodies interpret it as a sweet food. Secondly, those same sweeteners can increase our cravings for other sweet foods. Not good!

Irrespective of the rationale behind it, I have witnessed dozens of my clients lose weight at amazing rates once they kick their diet-drink habit. I'd strongly advise you avoid them too.

Alcohol

We've covered this already, but just to remind you: alcohol is a refined carbohydrate; what's more, calories derived from it will be burned up before calories from fat and glucose. Put frankly:

> The more booze that passes your lips, the more fat will sit on your hips!

However, as the Pyramid plan is for life I will be realistic. If you enjoy the odd tipple on special occasions, choose wisely and, if possible, limit this luxury to high-carb days only.

Take a look at the tables in Chapter 16. Note that drinks such as lager, bitter and liqueurs are high GI and must absolutely be avoided. Wines and spirits are mostly low GI and can be enjoyed in moderation. If you've been a beer drinker up until now, make the switch before it's too late. Excess weight around the midriff is notoriously hard to shift, and a huge price to pay for a quick drink down the local. If this has become a part of your daily routine, find an active hobby in which to invest your spare time and money such as golf, tennis, gardening or simply joining the gym. Your body will thank you for it!

CUTTING DOWN ON THE BOOZE

Cutting down on alcohol long-term can be difficult for the best of us. Think it won't hinder your weight-loss? Think again!

Meet 27-year-old Debbie South, a sales-support assistant from Essex. Debbie had always been slightly overweight, but says the weight really started creeping on between the ages of 19 and 25. Debbie would work at a desk all week, then party all weekend, indulging in wine, beer, cocktails and shots.

Debbie says: 'I'd always been a chubby child, and by the time I reached my late teens I'd become quite self-conscious. I started going clubbing with my friends and always thought going out straight from work and skipping dinner would help me to slim down, because I was surviving on fluids. I'd go out most Friday nights, get up late Saturday, have a couple of slices of toast or a sandwich and be straight out again to the next party.

'Month by month, year by year, I got bigger and bigger and just couldn't understand why. The bigger I got, the less I'd eat and the more I'd make up for this at the bar. I'd drink beer, wine, cocktails, whatever the tipple of the town was on that particular night. I wasn't an alcoholic, I could quite easily have enjoyed cosy nights in with a cup of tea, but I feared if I did this I'd end up eating.

'I reached my heaviest in March 2010, when I hit 19st 2lbs and wore a size 22. I felt gross and my party lifestyle wasn't even fun anymore. That's when one of my friends introduced me to Danni and she explained it was the alcohol that was causing me to gain so much weight.

'I started the Pyramid Diet right away and gave up booze totally. It was a real relief being able to eat proper meals and snacks throughout the day without being terrified I was going to pile on the pounds. Being able to enjoy food and not feel guilty about it was a novelty, and learning that in actual fact I wasn't eating *enough* came as a real surprise. When you're very overweight, you do tend to worry about what people will think when they see you eating. Looking back, I think this was another factor contributing to my weight-gain. I'd be too scared to eat at my desk in case people thought, "Oh look, the overweight girl is eating again."

'The best thing about adopting the Pyramid Diet is the fact you can still eat bread and pasta. These are both things I love, and never would have dreamed I could eat and still lose weight. I've become quite a chef and really enjoy experimenting with healthy ingredients when I get the time.

'In February 2011, I joined the gym and have also taken part in some sponsored runs. I adore working out and cannot believe I missed out on it for all those years! I'm currently 14st 2lbs, meaning I've lost a total of 5 stone in 18 months, but I'm not finished yet! I've gone from a size 22 to a size 14 and can now shop in high-street shops with the girls without feeling left out.

'So long as you are sensible and control your portion sizes, it's really hard to go wrong with the Pyramid method. I think the reason it worked for me is because I knew I was allowed to eat my favourite foods and as a result I didn't crave processed junk

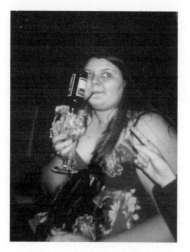

(left) Debbie at her heaviest, out partying in 2010
(right) Running the Race for Life in 2011

or huge portions. I feel fantastic, people say I look great and I've never been happier! I have the odd glass of wine on special occasions, but now that I know the impact alcohol can have on my waistline it's just not worth drinking regularly. I'd sooner have my new body than a measly cocktail any day!'

Hopefully, Debbie's story has inspired you to moderate or eliminate your alcohol intake in favour of a sustainable body you are proud of. Alcohol does damage on the inside as well as the outside, remember, so I really cannot stress the importance of this enough.

THE GOOD NEWS ABOUT BOOZE

If you do decide to drink socially from time to time, red wine should be your preferred option. Here are a few welcome reasons:

- Moderate, regular consumption of red wine may help to prevent coronary heart disease by reducing levels of LDL (bad cholesterol), whilst boosting HDL (good cholesterol).
- Two small glasses of red wine (total 250ml), consumed with a meal, can help to lower post-meal blood pressure in hypertensive people.
- Red wine reduces the risk of kidney stones.
- The alcohol and polyphenols in red wine can help to maintain healthy blood vessels by promoting the formation of nitric oxide, the key chemical in enabling the blood vessels to relax, and thus preventing hardening of the arteries.

- Resveratrol, a polyphenol found in red wine, produces neuroprotective effects, and can lower the risk of developing Alzheimer's disease.

You've had a lot to absorb in this chapter, but hopefully you've learned a lot too! Before we move on, I'd like you to meet Renny, a 27-year-old musician who barely knew the words 'vegetables' or 'fish' before embarking on the Pyramid Diet.

RENNY'S STORY

'I'm in a band and regularly tour the country singing and playing the guitar. I'd normally wake up around 2pm, eat a few bags of crisps and a few cans of diet drinks and write music all day. Come the evening, the band would often have a gig, in which case I'd eat whatever the venue had to offer, along with a few beers to wash it all down. I've always played football once a week, but was beginning to struggle due to excess weight and lack of fitness.

'In 2010, I decided it was time to do something about my weight, as it had started to spiral out of control and I was too physically exhausted to perform on stage to the best of my ability. I contacted Danni and she put me on the Pyramid Diet right away. At the time, I wasn't too impressed, because I had to bin the fizzy drinks and I was told to get up by 10am every day and go for a run. It felt like the middle of the night to me!

'After a couple of weeks, I began getting into the swing of things, and was enjoying waking up to a healthy breakfast and taking regular snacks throughout the day. I cut back on beer dramatically at gigs and would always make sure I had dinner before leaving the house, or simply decline the greasy chips and kebabs I used to indulge in.

'For me, the Pyramid Diet just seems to make sense and fits in with my lifestyle really well. The weight literally fell off me, and whilst I don't weigh myself I think I lost around 3 stone in the space of 2–3 months. Not once did I go hungry and not once did I crave a bag of crisps or a fizzy drink. I've even started doing a bit of cooking, much to Mum's delight! The rigidity offered by the diet is perfect for me, because I know I will never ever go back to my old ways again. My singing has improved and I'm now the star of my football team!'

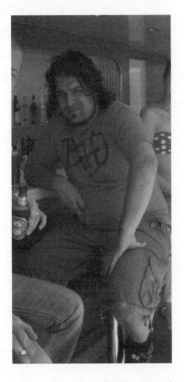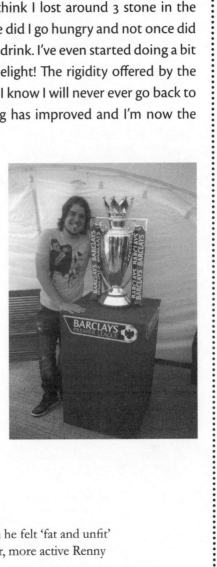

(*left*) Renny when he felt 'fat and unfit'
(*right*) A slimmer, more active Renny

You are now about to embark on building the foundations of *your* Pyramid. So wave goodbye to that excess weight for ever and say hello to a new way of life!

6. Planning Your Pyramid

So far, I've explained to you the fundamentals of the Pyramid Diet and the dietary rules you must adhere to in order to reap the benefits. You'll hopefully have acquired some invaluable knowledge on the mechanics of carb-cycling, and will be looking forward to saying hello to the body you deserve.

In Chapters 7–9, we'll be taking an in-depth look at the three days which collectively make up the Pyramid: high-carb, low-carb and no-carb. But before we move on to this important structural analysis, let's lay some firm foundations for your own personal Pyramid.

Your Priorities

We all have our favourite foods we simply couldn't live without. Whether you've a passion for pasta or go barmy for bread, be honest with yourself, it's no good trying to deny these culinary desires to yourself for ever. Whilst not all foods are permissible on the Pyramid Diet, there are easy compromises and surprisingly small adaptations that can be made in order to transform your body and your mind. These changes can also help to alter the neural pathways leading from your brain to your body, which tell you you're full up and prevent you from overeating.

Jot down the foods you feel you'd be hard pushed to go

without. Do you enjoy an Italian pasta once a week with friends? Or perhaps you frequent the local Chinese takeaway with a loved one? Whatever your food faux pas, the Pyramid Diet has you covered! You may need to refer to the tables in Part Five from time to time for suitable swaps, but your mind and tastebuds will soon get used to these marginal adaptations, and the rewards will be both visually and mentally encouraging.

As we've seen, it's not uncommon for diets to dictate an initial period of abstinence from certain foods or drinks, after which you are allowed to slowly wean yourself back on to them. Nine times out of ten, this method will just reintroduce the unwanted weight and sugar cravings you thought you'd disposed of. Now, I'm not going to ask you to live a life of misery, where parties are a thing of the past and restaurants go out of business. Ever heard the saying 'A little of what you fancy does you good'? Well, it's absolutely true! Dedication does not have to mean deprivation.

Decided what's most important to you? Great! Now you're ready to start cementing the foundations of a lifetime.

Your Essentials

Now you're ready to start building your Pyramid, piece by piece, day by day. Of course, once you are familiar with the carb-cycling routine and the way in which the Pyramid works, you'll be able to improvize on the spot when you're out and about, on holiday, or simply don't feel like cooking. Until then, start off with something slightly more structured and organized. This will give you the rigidity you need as part of the learning curve, ensuring you get off to a faultless start.

You will find it useful to compile an 'Essentials' list of food with which to fill your kitchen cupboards and fridge, staple foods which will form the foundations of your diet and can be used in a variety of meals and snacks throughout the day or are handy to pop in your bag and eat on the go. Examples of these foods are:

Good Carbs

- Fruit (choose wisely from low GI options in the tables)
- Green fibrous vegetables such as broccoli and spinach
- Sweet potatoes (ideal for mashing, baking or turning into wedges)
- Oats (can be eaten for breakfast or used in a variety of tasty recipes)
- Wholewheat pasta (a great treat on high-carb days)
- Unsweetened popcorn (for when you can't resist a nibble in front of a DVD)

No Carb/High Protein

- Eggs
- Low-fat cheddar or cottage cheese
- Natural, unsweetened, 'live' yoghurt
- Soya and skimmed milk (in moderation)
- Unsweetened or homemade vegetable soups
- Unsweetened nuts and seeds to nibble on
- Fish
- Meat, poultry and game (lean cuts only)

Good Extras

- Salad items such as lettuce, cucumber and radishes
- Your favourite fresh and dried herbs
- A selection of condiments such as sugar-free tomato ketchup, extra-virgin olive oil, vinegar, black pepper and spices
- A good variety of black, green and herbal teas

Tightening Your Belt

Protein is an essential requirement for all three days on the Pyramid Diet and meat can be expensive. Don't let this put you off. The Pyramid Diet can be followed successfully, regardless of your food budget.

It's a common misconception that junk food is cheaper than quality, fresh produce. This is simply not the case. Browse the confectionary aisles of a newsagent's and you'll notice a standard chocolate bar now costs 70–80 pence. An apple, on the other hand, is only likely to set you back 40–50 pence. A lunchtime 'meal deal', something which is widely available from various food chains, typically costs around £5 and consists of a soft drink, a sandwich and a bag of crisps, piece of fruit or a dessert. This may seem like a bargain when those familiar afternoon hunger pangs are persistently causing your tummy to rumble and your boss wants you back at your desk within twenty minutes. After all, it's quick, cheap and provides you with a 'healthy option' compared to other fast foods. And yet the 'meal deal' is *not* fantastic value for money and definitely not wise for your waist.

And how much money do you splash out during a typical week on takeaways, alcohol, sweet treats and other non-essential food items? How many times do you stop off at your favourite coffee outlet, only to hand over £3 for a cardboard cup filled with milk or water and a spoonful of caffeine? Add up the money spent on these luxuries and you'll soon discover you have plenty of spare change to spend on products which will put a dent in your waistline, not your wallet.

Building the foundations of the Pyramid is partially about making lifestyle changes, taking a new approach to food and drink in order to filter out unwanted sugar and additives and cut down on unnecessary spending. The following table illustrates a handful of price comparisons between common 'bad' food choices and suggested Pyramid-approved swaps, which are great for stocking up on, or making a note of before you set sail.*

Bad Choice	Price	Swap for	Price	Saving
Hovis soft white bread 800g	£1.15	Tesco Finest rustic multi-grain sliced bread 800g	£1.00	15p
Tesco Finest green veg selection 260g (with added butter & salt)	£2.65	Tesco green beans 92p for 220g + Tesco hand-shelled garden peas £1.40 for 170g	£2.32	33p, with veg to spare!
Walkers cheese & onion crisps, 6 pack	£1.48	Tesco Market-value apple tray, 6 pack	99p	49p
Skippy extra crunchy peanut butter, 340g	£2.26	Whole Earth crunchy original peanut butter with no added sugar, 340g	£1.95	31p
Asda butter-basted chicken breast joint	£6 per kg	Asda British free-range whole chicken	£4.28 per kg	£1.72 per kg

* Obviously prices will vary over time and location. These prices were taken from various stores around the UK at the time of going to press.

These Pyramid-approved swaps demonstrate you do not have to spend more to eat well.

Yet another strategy to keep your costs down would be to cut the amount of meat you eat every week, replacing that protein with vegetarian sources. See Chapter 10 for lots of suggestions if you want to try this.

Making Your Plan

When you think about it, without some form of structure in our lives, we'd all fall apart. From taking a shower, to going to bed when we're tired, we routinely do most things like clockwork without giving them a second thought, yet they all have their own time slots allocated throughout the day. So why should our diets be any different? Why is it we leave ourselves unprepared at mealtimes, then when hunger strikes we grab the first sandwich or bag of crisps we see from the petrol station as a last-minute pick-me-up? If we placed more importance on mealtimes, that last-minute dash to the lunch line would become a thing of the past, leaving us more time to relax and doing wonders for the waistband.

Since I first started prescribing the Pyramid Diet to my clients, the questions I have most frequently encountered are 'How am I supposed to remember which day is which?' and 'What happens if I have a meal to go to and eat too many carbs on a low-carb or no-carb day?' We will see how to make the Pyramid fit into your lifestyle in Part Four, but there are some essential sacrifices to be made (at least initially) if you are serious about taking your body by storm. Once you have prioritized your favourite foods and laid the foundations for the road ahead, it's time to add structure to your new way of eating. As human beings, we only respond well to structure if we are also given a degree of flexibility and vice-versa. Whilst there is room for some shift in the Pyramid Diet, the fundamentals must be adhered to if you are to see real results.

So sit down and think about your week, and plan ahead! You know you'll need to eat regular meals, plus snack on the correct foods in between, so plan your menus for the week before you shop, and set aside time to make your packed lunch plus snacks every day.

Before long, you will be able to select the relevant amount of carbohydrates and barely have to think twice about totting things up. As with any new diet plan though, there is some beginner's groundwork to be done. The great thing is, once you become familiar with the carb content of certain foods and learn to make sensible swaps, you'll never have to worry about those fancy, fad diets again.

Setting Your Goal

A quick word about setting your personal goal: I always advise clients to use a target dress size, waist size, or their favourite pair of under-sized jeans as a goal, *not* body-weight. Once you achieve this goal and step on the scales, you will be reassured by what they tell you. Weighing yourself day in, day out (especially when carb-cycling) is anyway not advisable. The slightest disappointment can cause setbacks and, as we'll see later on, it is not just body-weight I want you to concern yourself with.

Know Your Limits

Before we look at the limits to your carb intake in detail, it's important to understand that it's the *net*-carb content of foods that is used. This can be worked out by subtracting a food's fibre content from its total carb content.

Total Carbs − Fibre = Net Carbs

The relevant figures should be marked on a food's packaging, but you'll also find the most common foods listed in the tables in Part Five.

Your Weight and Your Carb Limits

The upper limit for net carbs on Day 1, high-carb day, is 1g per lb of body-weight. So if you weigh 200lb you can eat up to 200g of carbs. That figure is halved for low-carb day, so for the same person it would be 100g. The limit for no-carb day is 20g, whatever weight you are.

As your body weight depreciates, you will need to adjust your carb limits accordingly. You may become accustomed to chomping your way through 200g of net carbs on high-carb day, then, on weighing yourself a few weeks later, discover your weight has dropped to 180lbs, making your new carb limit 180g.

I'm often asked when and how frequently the carb limit should be adjusted. After all, if we weighed ourselves every day (which some of us just can't resist) and saw the weight come off ounce by ounce, it would be an almost impossible and certainly very complex task to continually drop your carb limit one gram at a time.

For these reasons, I advise you to weigh yourself only once every two weeks and only ever on the same type of day. You will typically be heavier after a high-carb day than you will after low- and no-carb days, because you will be holding more water. If you want to weigh yourself weekly then be my guest, but you will then be obliged to drop your maximum carb limit more frequently. Two weeks is not sufficient time for maximum limits to soar too high above your new body weight, yet it is a short enough period to ensure you adjust these limits before it's too late. (Of course you aim to reach a happy and sustainable weight eventually, at which point you will no longer be losing weight. Once this happens, we will work together in Chapter 12, 'The Pyramid for Life', to find the upper-carb limit that suits you.)

Below is an example of the carb limits for a 200lb Pyramid dieter with a target weight of 160lbs. You will see their upper-carb limits are adjusted in increments until they reach their goal weight. (Please note: this is a hypothetical example only and not intended to be a guide to expected weight-loss.)

Weight	Week 1 200lb	Week 3 190lb	Week 5 180lb	Week 7 170lb	Week 9 160lb
High-carb day	200g	190g	180g	170g	160g
Low-carb day	100g	95g	90g	85g	80g
No-carb day	20g	20g	20g	20g	20g

The dieter in this example would continue carb consumption according to the upper limit at their goal weight (in this case 160g of net carbs on a high-carb day). If they continued to lose weight against their will, they would use one of the variables set out in Chapter 12 to find the exact carb limit or Pyramid pattern which works for them at their new weight.

For now, you just need to concern yourself with reaching your perfect weight, and this is done by adhering to the default carb limits and three-day cycle.

Most wholegrain, unrefined carbs are Pyramid-approved, but be sure to check the tables to see which ones come with the lowest GI or GL. In some cases, you will find you have a choice between two options, yet one has a marginally lower GI or is higher in protein. When these circumstances arise, always opt for the more healthy of the two. For example, granary and wholemeal bread (without added sugar) are both allowed, but the grains in granary bread brings the glycaemic load down, making it the better option. Similarly, it is wiser to consume pasta with a meat or Quorn sauce than a simple tomato or oil-based sauce, because the protein will bring down the glycaemic load of the entire meal.

Bear in mind it does not matter which day of the cycle you are on, or how many carbs you are limited to, you will still benefit from keeping the glycaemic load of your meals as low as possible to prevent insulin spikes. And when choosing wholegrain products, remember, don't be swayed by sneaky advertizing or natural-looking packaging. Just because something is 'wholegrain' does not mean it is free from added sugar. When you are stocking up your cupboards, it is imperative you scrutinize every label to be sure you are not buying sugar.

The Protein Goals

Once you've worked out your own starting carb limits, you'll need to calculate how much protein you should aim to eat every day. It is extremely important that you try to consume at least 1g of protein per lb of body weight, and that you try to include protein in each meal. On low- and no-carb days, you may well find your protein intake is higher than on high-carb days, when you will be getting more of your daily energy intake from foods such as wholegrains. Make good use of foods such as nuts and seeds on low- and no-carb days, as well as eating plenty of green vegetables. Your digestive system would not thank you if you survived on meat alone every third day.

Diets that eliminate carbohydrates entirely are infamous for expecting you to consume vast amounts of protein in what can sometimes be limitless quantities. The Pyramid Diet sets a protein goal because it appreciates the importance of protein. However, don't be tempted to gorge yourself on steak after steak on no-carb day, as excessive protein consumption can lead to metabolic acidosis. This condition occurs when there is too much acid in your body, or when your kidneys are not effectively removing acid and is particularly prevalent in those following diets that send their bodies into a state of ketosis, where fat is used for energy instead of carbohydrates (because there are no glycogen stores in the body). This excess acidity can also lead to loss of calcium in the bones.

Because protein cannot be consumed in limitless quantities, this effectively makes the Pyramid Diet a calorie-cycling diet as well as a carb-cycling one. You *will* consume fewer calories on no-carb day than you will on high- and low-carb day. You will not have to think about this; it will just come naturally. The Pyramid doesn't set an upper protein limit; instead, I ask you to make sensible choices. One steak for dinner is fine. Two steaks would be excessive. Don't go hungry but never stuff yourself.

One more thing before we move on. You will undoubtedly consume more fats on no-carb day than you will on high-carb day. This is intentional and will *not* make you fat. As you know, at 9 calories per gram, fat has a higher energy content than carbohydrates and protein but you will need these calories on no-carb day, as you will be receiving no more than 80 calories (from 20g) from carbohydrates.

Combining These Principles

With all of this in mind, let's take a look at some facts and figures and apply them to different body-weights. How much food should you be eating to maintain your current body-weight, without losing or gaining weight? There is a formula we can use to determine the approximate number of calories needed on a daily basis. This formula does not take physical activity into consideration, however, so those of us who lead active lifestyles will need more energy than what this calculation will determine.

The Pyramid Diet does not count calories, but it does help to talk about them in order to better understand the construction of the Pyramid. A balanced, nutritious diet is essential for weight-loss, or for maintaining a slender figure. But the bottom line is, if we consume more calories than we burn, we will gain weight.

We need to burn approximately 3,500 calories more than we consume to lose 1lb through catabolism. Conversely, if we eat more calories than we need, we will gain approximately 1lb for every 3,500 calories too many. You can work out how many calories you need to maintain your current body-weight by using the formula below.

- Find out your body-weight in pounds.
- Multiply this by 10 (so, if you weigh 150lbs, then
  150 × 10 = 1,500).

 – Add your body-weight to that figure (1,500 + 150 = 1,650).

And there's your answer in three simple steps – if you weigh 150lbs, you'll need approximately 1,650 calories per day to maintain your body-weight. (Remember, if you exercise, you'll need more!)

Let's assume they do want to lose weight. In the case of the 150lb dieter aiming to lose 28lbs (2 stone), they would need to create a deficit over time of 28 × 3,500 calories which comes to 98,000 calories. Most diets work by cutting calories to, for example, 1,150 per day, thus creating an energy deficit and sending the body into catabolism. Over the course of a week, this dieter would therefore lose at least 1lb in weight.

But as you've already learned, the Pyramid Diet alternates between anabolism and catabolism, which essentially means you must not survive on a calorie-deficient diet every day if you want to continue to lose weight and keep your metabolism fired up. Based on Pyramid principles, let's now revisit the 150lb dieter to see how their diet would look from a Pyramid perspective. Remember that carbs and protein contain 4 calories per gram, whilst fat contains 9.

High-Carb Day

Maximum carb intake = 150g	= 600 calories
Minimum protein intake = 150g	= 600 calories
Approximate fat intake = 60g	= 540 calories
Additional calories from fibrous vegetables	= 100 calories
Total	**= 1,840 calories**

This comes in at 190 above the body-weight maintenance threshold of 1,650 calories per day for a 150lb person. However, this is based on the minimum protein intake and a reasonably low fat intake. In reality, the number of calories consumed on high-carb day could be as high as 2,200. You needn't worry about this; it's a positive thing and a crucial component of the Pyramid pattern.

On a low-carb day, the 150lb person's carbohydrate consumption is halved to 75g. On a no-carb day, the maximum number of calories anyone can consume from carbohydrates is 80. Below is an example of how a no-carb day may look for the same person weighing 150lbs.

No-Carb Day

Maximum carb intake = 20g	= 80 calories
Minimum protein intake = 150g	= 600 calories
Approximate fat intake = 70g	= 630 calories
Additional calories from fibrous vegetables	= 150 calories
Total	**= 1,460 calories**

Although the protein and fat intake on no-carb day may be slightly higher than shown in the example above, you can see that a 150lb person would be creating a deficit of around 190 calories for that day by following this formula – without even taking exercise into consideration. This means they would be in a state of catabolism and draw on the glycogen reserves their body had set aside from high-carb day to use as energy. Once these reserves have been depleted, their system will eat into fat stores, meaning they will lose weight.

Understanding Portion Sizes

One of the biggest obstacles we face when trying to lose weight is knowing how much food we're supposed to eat in one sitting. We've all heard the saying 'You are what you eat', and to a large extent this is absolutely right. However, you are also how *much* you eat. Not only does the glycaemic load of a meal increase the larger that meal is, the net-carb and calorie content also increase.

Think about it: if you ate 100 apples, 3kg of granary bread and 20 chickens, you'd put on weight! OK, this is an extreme example, but even that extra spoonful of rice or additional piece of bread could be what's stopping you from losing weight. Too many of us now believe we are *what* we eat and think we can go overboard on the portion sizes. I believe very low-carb diets are partially to blame, as they lead us to believe we can eat endless quantities of protein-rich foods and not gain an ounce. Think back to Chapter 2, when we spoke about metabolism. One of the fundamental components of an effective metabolism is catabolism, which only dominates when we have an energy deficit from consuming fewer calories than we need.

You are unlikely to go catabolic on a high-carb day, and I don't want you to because this keeps your body guessing. However, you still need to watch your portions to avoid gaining fat. Eating more calories than you need to avoid a deficit is one thing; binge-eating is another. Eating until you are stuffed will have no nutritional or dietary benefit whatsoever, and will hinder your weight-loss, even if you only do it on a high-carb day. I am fairly confident you will not fall into this trap, because the upper net-carb limits set by the Pyramid will not allow you to do so. However, there is one little hole in the net, which is all too easy to fall through . . .

Restaurants and Takeaways

Some of you may be fortunate enough to find restaurants and takeaway outlets that serve brown rice or wholewheat pasta. Others will simply enjoy nibbling on wholegrain bread rolls from the bread basket with their meal. Either way, when you are not in control of the kitchen, matters can easily get out of hand. I suggest sticking to a maximum of one bread roll with your meal and asking the waiter to limit your rice or pasta portion to 125g. This quantity makes for a satiating but sensible serving size, and they really won't mind you asking.

The worst culprits are buffet-style restaurants and all-you-can-eat chains. If you do choose to visit these places, use the self-selection element to your advantage, rather than letting it lead to plate overload. There are normally plenty of healthy dishes to choose from, such as steamed vegetables, salads, chicken skewers and mussels. Just be on your guard where sauces are concerned, as many restaurant sauces contain saturated fats or thickening agents such as cornflour. As a rule, black-bean style sauces make for a more healthy choice than sweet sauces, which typically contain added sugar. If you order plain food such as meat and pepper skewers from the hot plate, ask the chef if they stock soy sauce. Used in moderation, it adds flavour without the sugar or calories found in most other sauces.

Another flavoursome addition to food of any cuisine is garlic. If you are a fan of its taste, it is well worth asking that it be added to restaurant food. Garlic suffers from a bad reputation in the breath department, but in my view its benefits outweigh its pungency. The many benefits of eating garlic regularly include reduced cholesterol, improved cardiovascular health and prevention and treatment of colds. If you're offended by the taste or smell of fresh garlic, why not try taking an odourless garlic supplement?

MIGUEL SAYS …

'I recently had a client come to me who was following a strict diet given to him by a dietician, and initially he lost a lot of weight. By the time he approached me for fitness advice, his weight-loss had plateaued, and he could only assume it was because he was not doing any exercise. I took a look at his diet sheet and instantly knew there was another reason, because at almost 16st and just 5'4" tall, he'd have needed substantially more calories each day to maintain his weight than he claimed he was eating.

I noticed pasta featured heavily on his diet plan. I asked if he ate out in restaurants very often – he did almost every night. It turned out he'd been following everything the dietician had advised him to the letter, but hadn't thought to check the portion sizes he was being served. I spoke to the chef at the restaurant he ate in most frequently, and asked him to limit the portion size of my client's pasta to just 100g. The chef obliged, and from then on the weight came off at a much faster rate.'

Home Cooking

Whilst it is easier to implement portion control in our own kitchens, where there are other members of the family in the house, some of us run into trouble. Picture this scenario:

You serve yourself and the rest of the family 125g brown rice with a grilled chicken breast and broccoli at dinner time on a high-carb day. You give yourself a pat on the back for following the Pyramid plan so perfectly, and collect up the empty dinner plates. Except the kids' plates aren't quite empty. They've left a little chicken and rice that they couldn't quite manage to eat, because they're more concerned about going to meet their friends. You pick up the fork and take one more mouthful of rice. 'Waste not, want not', you think to yourself. That's what your mother always taught you and it saves throwing away good food. Before you know it, you've eaten 200g of brown rice – well over the allocated 125g.

So you've decided what your priorities are, chosen your 'Essentials', thought about how you're going to plan your week, and understood a bit about your limits and portion sizes. Now it's time to start your life-changing Pyramid Diet!

PART THREE

The Pyramid Diet

7. Day 1: High-Carb Day

Most of you will find Day 1 of the three-day cycle – high-carb day – by far the easiest and most enjoyable. Your carb intake will be relatively high and you should feel comfortably satisfied all day long. As you know by now, throwing in a high-carb day every three days will keep your body guessing. High-carb days raise the body's insulin levels and fill your glycogen stores, keeping your metabolism burning efficiently and staving off muscle catabolism. There's no need to feel guilty – after all, carbohydrates are the only form of fuel used by the brain, so you're also stocking up on a good healthy dose of brain food.

We've talked about the limits in the previous chapter, but I suspect you're still a bit baffled, having probably never studied the carbohydrate content of foods in depth before. Don't worry, I promise once you become accustomed to this it'll become second nature. You're not being asked to count calories, or even count points. Carb contents are something which take a little getting used to, but that is all.

And as we touched on, it is the *net*-carb figure you will be working with, not the total. In some cases, fibre will already have been deducted from the total carb count on the food label and won't be listed separately. If this happens, just go by the total carb count. But in any case, you will only be able to consume a limited range of carbohydrate-based products, listed in Part Five. Just refer to this for guidance if you're unsure on the net-carb content of a specific food.

As a means of getting you started, have a look at the sample table below, which details the approximate number of grams of net carbs in certain popular, allowable foods.[*]

Carbohydrate	Serving	Net Carbs
Sweet potato	1 medium	25g
Granary bread	1 slice	12.5g
Oats (rolled)	40g	20g
Quinoa	1 tbsp	25g
Polenta	100g	15g
Brown rice	100g	30g
Wholewheat spaghetti	100g	30g
Couscous	100g	20g
Muesli (unsweetened)	30g	30g
Wholegrain rice cakes	2	12g
Corn-on-the-cob	1 medium	15g
Carrot	100g	5g
Beetroot	50g	5g
Butternut squash	130g	10g

Let's work on the basis you weigh 140lbs, so your carb allowance for the day is 140g. If you choose to have 40g oats for breakfast, containing 20g net carbs, you have 120g of your carb allowance remaining. You may then opt for a granary-bread sandwich for lunch, which would give you a further 25g of net carbs. Even if your dinner then included a sweet potato at 25g net carbs, you would still have a whopping 50g of your

* For easy calculations, some quantities have been rounded up or down. In packaged products, quantities may vary according to manufacturer, so always check the label.

carb allowance remaining for meals or snacks in between. So as you can see, the Pyramid Diet is all about choosing the right carbs to put into your body, not cutting them out of your life.

A Typical High-Carb Day

So what does a typical high-carb day look like? Of course it is entirely up to you what you choose to cook up, but sometimes you may be confined to the office chair or committed to a meal with friends or colleagues. If this is the case, don't find yourself in a panic. There are plenty of things you can eat which thankfully are now widely available in popular cafés, restaurants and supermarkets. Many of the products on the Pyramid carb menu are listed in their natural state and all you have to do is choose suitable toppings, fillings or accompaniments.

The following menu is an example of what a typical 140lb man or woman might eat on a high-carb day:

	Net Carbs
Meal 1: 40g oats flavoured with a dash of cinnamon	20g
Meal 2: 2 wholegrain rice cakes with natural peanut butter	20g
Meal 3: Chicken breast with 100g brown rice and salad	30g
Meal 4: Large banana	30g
Meal 5: Salmon, broccoli and sweet potato	25g
Meal 6: Fruit salad	15g
Total	**140g**

Whilst in this example you would have eaten the maximum quantity of carbs available to you, this is not essential. If you only consume 120g or even 100g on high-carb day, that is fine. So long as you feel satisfied and don't find yourself craving more of these foods, your body is telling you you've had enough. Neither is it imperative that every meal contains carbs. If for Meal 3, for example, you just wanted to have chicken and vegetables without rice, that would be absolutely fine. The high-carb allowance is the maximum allowed, not the goal.

Eating Out and On the Go

No matter what your work or social commitments, all three days on the Pyramid Diet are designed to make your life easy. The following menu is an example of a high-carb day for someone on the go, who doesn't have time to cook, and is perhaps eating from an office canteen in the day, then going out for dinner in the evening. As you can see, despite eating a wide variety of foods all day, you would still have 40g of net carbs to play with, which could be used for something like an alcoholic drink.

Once again, this is based on an individual of 140lbs. You will need to vary quantities according to your own body-weight.

	Net Carbs
Meal 1: 2 slices of brown toast with natural peanut butter	30g
Meal 2: Small fruit-salad pot	20g
Meal 3: Tuna and bean salad pot	10g
Meal 4: Natural Greek yoghurt pot	5g
Meal 5: Smoked salmon platter with brown bread	25g
Meal 6: Sirloin steak with vegetables, mushrooms and tomatoes	10g
Total	**100g**

In the above sequence, Meal 5 would be your starter to your evening dinner. Meal 3 would typically be your lunch from a local café or your office canteen. Things like fruit-salad pots, bean-based salads and natural yoghurt are all widely available in even the smallest outlets. If you're at a fish restaurant or choosing from an à la carte menu, just ask for the dish to come without potatoes or white rice. Even on a high-carb day, these are not acceptable foods, remember, and you don't have to have carbs at every meal. Some restaurants do offer brown rice, but always check before ordering.

If you're at a pasta restaurant or pizzeria, the Pyramid can present slightly more of a challenge, but it's still easy once you know how. Some restaurants serve wholemeal pizza bases or wholewheat pasta. If this is the case, go for it and enjoy something from their usual menu. If they insist on feeding diners products made with white flour, don't give in to the temptation and order a 16″ meat feast! There are plenty of other tasty options found in a typical Italian-style restaurant. The following list will give you some ideas:

Starters

— Seared scallops with butternut squash
— Moules marinières
— Garlic and tomato tiger prawns
— Goat's cheese salad
— Beef carpaccio

Mains

— Chicken in a white wine and mushroom sauce with wild brown rice

- Fillet steak with side order of mushrooms and vegetables
- Fillet of salmon with side order of vegetables
- Chicken pesto salad
- Seared tuna with salad or vegetables
- Pan-fried cod marinated with olives, tomatoes and asparagus

Desserts

- Fresh fruit salad
- Strawberries (no sugar or cream)

Side orders

- Wholemeal bread rolls
- Olives
- Olive oil and pesto-based dips

Drinks

- Espresso
- Tea and Coffee
- Water
- A maximum of two alcoholic drinks (but try to avoid this)

Remember, avoid white bread, white pasta, white pizza bases, breaded chicken, lasagne, white rice and croutons.

That's the Italian dealt with, but how would you tackle a Chinese? Whether you're in a restaurant or ordering a take-away, Chinese food tends to be packed with refined carbs. As always, though, any cuisine is possible on the Pyramid Diet.

Here is a selection of dishes you could order from a Chinese restaurant:

Starters

— Mussels in black-bean sauce
— Chicken satay
— Plain spare ribs (no BBQ sauce)
— Pork satay
— Clear soups

Mains

— Beef/chicken/pork in black-bean sauce with steamed vegetables
— Beef/chicken/pork stir-fry with beansprouts (no noodles or rice) and soy sauce
— Steamed fish with steamed vegetables and soy sauce or ginger
— Steamed tofu with steamed vegetables and soy sauce or ginger
— Walnut chicken
— Szechuan prawns
— Curry beef or chicken (without rice)

Desserts

— Go for something fruity and ask for it to be served with no added sugar. Many Chinese restaurants serve lychee- or pear-based desserts which you can enjoy without the sugar-laden ice cream which often comes with it.

Avoid BBQ Sauce, sweet and sour sauce, hoisin sauce, white rice, white noodles, prawn crackers, battered chicken or pork balls, spring rolls and thick soups.

Treats and Snacks

Now that you're aware of just some of the delicious dishes you can have on high-carb day, I want to introduce you to some suitable treats and snacks for when you're on the go. The recipes for these and lots more tasty nibbles are in Chapter 15.

Tasty treats

- Chocolate protein-packed brownies
- Organic chocolate cookies
- Fresh fruit and natural yoghurt
- Delicious healthy cheesecake
- Sugar-free jelly
- Pyramid almond-butter cookies

Snacks

- Natural yoghurt
- Low GI dried fruit with nuts
- Oat bar (unsweetened)
- Low-fat cheese portion (30g)
- Beef jerky
- Wholegrain rice cakes with turkey slices or nut butter
- Carrot and celery sticks (mixed)

— Fresh fruit
— Chicken satay sticks

Protein on High-Carb Day

Remember, you need to aim for at least 1g of protein per lb of body-weight. This applies every day, not just on high-carb day, and it's better to stagger your intake through the day. If you include protein in every meal you will find your protein target much more attainable than if you eat toast for breakfast, wholewheat pasta for lunch and leave the protein until the evening.

If you're still struggling, get yourself a low-calorie, low-carb, lactose-free protein shake to supplement your diet. These come in a variety of delicious flavours and taste just like a milkshake. Mix with water and for best results, drink just before you go to bed at night, or after exercise. Depending on the brand you choose, this simple addition to your diet will pack in about 45g of extra protein per day.

Exercise

The benefits of regular exercise are discussed at length in Chapter 13. Whether you're a beginner or a keen athlete, you'll soon be able to adapt your fitness programme to give it maximum compatibility with the Pyramid Diet. Hand in hand, diet and exercise are always more powerful than diet alone.

If you already exercise regularly, high-carb days are not great days to do a cardiovascular activity such as running or cycling. This is because insulin inhibits fat-burning. Leave the cardio to the low-carb and no-carb days, but feel free to perform resistance (or weight-bearing) exercise if you want to work out.

Don't Drop the High-Carb Day!

Ever since I first started prescribing the Pyramid Diet to overweight clients, I have been asked countless times whether it is OK to skip the high-carb day for fear of it slowing the weight-loss process. I live in hope that you have read, absorbed and accepted the science behind the Pyramid in Chapter 2, but nevertheless I acknowledge that a fair few of you may already be contemplating the same question. I know it is tempting to try to kick-start your weight-loss plan by cutting carbs. Remember, the Pyramid Diet uses carbohydrates to your advantage, to help you not only lose weight but keep it off. Your body will undergo internal as well as external changes, and skipping the high-carb day will not have the same positive outcome. Take note of the following facts, then (please!) never fear high-carb day again:

- The 'high-carb' day in the Pyramid Diet is actually relatively low-carb when compared with our typical eating patterns. It is only 'high' in comparison to the low-carb and no-carb days. The daily maximum dosage of 1g of net carbs per lb of body-weight is not high enough to allow you to over-eat these types of foods.
- High-carb day fires up your metabolism, helping your body to burn fat more efficiently.

- High-carb day helps to prevent sugar cravings, by allowing you to enjoy healthy, nutritious carbohydrates and saving you from the biscuit tin.
- In order to build a lean, shapely body and stay young, we need to dip into anabolism every now and then. A permanently catabolic (calorie-deficient) diet causes ageing and slows the metabolism. High-carb day allows for anabolism but prevents excessive bingeing.
- The Pyramid Diet is a programme for life. Can you honestly imagine spending the rest of your life without ever eating bread, pasta, rice or fruit again? There is only so long you can sustain a severely carb-restricted diet. The scales may reward you for the first few days, but they sure won't stay that way!

Whilst I am not advocating throwing food away, it is better off put in the fridge and saved for salads than gobbled up in one sitting.

One lovely lady who learned this the hard way was 35-year-old former beach-babe Sachaa Pattison, whom Miguel and I were fortunate enough to work with on *Bigger Than Britney*.

'When I was in my early twenties, I was living in my native Australia. I spent most of my days in a bikini and loved every minute of it. I was proud to show off my slender curves, and with my long blonde hair I was often likened to a Baywatch babe. Aged 27, I met a gorgeous English guy, to whom I am now married, and moved to the UK to be with him. I soon fell pregnant with our first child and we were overjoyed. The only problem was, I suffered from dreadful morning sickness and the only thing that

SACHAA'S STORY

seemed to prevent it was food. I decided I deserved to eat what-ever I wanted (I was pregnant after all) and soon started piling on the pounds. I put it down to the baby bump and didn't worry about it too much, until after the birth when I realized the excess fat I'd accrued wasn't going away.

'A few short months after giving birth to our first child, I fell pregnant again and the food cycle resumed. I made the decision to put worrying about my weight on the back burner until I'd had the baby. This was to be our last child (we'd always wanted two), so once this pregnancy was over I'd be able to focus on my figure.

'After the second birth, things were hectic looking after two young children. The weeks and months went by, until they got to the age they were sitting at the table eating solid foods. For me, that was when the real problems started. The kids would always leave leftovers on their plates, and I would always polish them off! Whilst I was making an effort to cook healthy meals for the family, I wasn't just eating mine, but most of the children's too. Slowly but surely I got bigger and bigger, until I reached my heaviest, at 12st 2lbs. That's when I applied to be on *Bigger Than Britney*, and I haven't looked back since.

'I now weigh 10st 4lbs and would ideally like to reach 9st, so I have a long way to go, but if I can achieve all of this in just 8 weeks and still enjoy my favourite foods, I know it won't be long before I reach my target weight. The Pyramid plan stops me picking at leftovers because I feel satisfied all the time, and each day is different! I no longer crave extra food and I can still eat out with friends and order from a standard menu. I'm never going back to my old ways now. I really thought I couldn't conquer my habits because I'm terrible at sticking to things. I know that if I can do it, anyone can!'

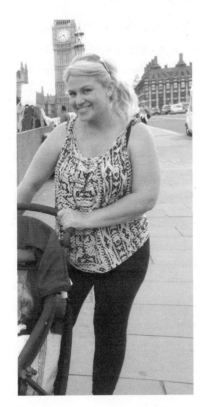
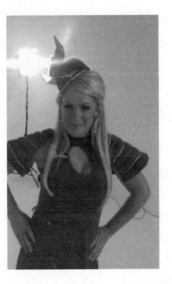

(left) Sachaa at her biggest
(right) Sachaa as a Pyramid dieter

Sachaa lost a total of 26lbs in just 8 weeks. She dropped from a dress size 16 to a size 12 and lost an incredible 6½ inches off her waist. Sachaa also followed my exercise programme to help build lean muscle and speed up fat-loss. The moral of this story?

Stick to One Plate or You'll Put On Weight!

Hopefully Sachaa's story has made you realize it's not too late to turn back the clock. Becoming a mum does not have to mean becoming a frump.

*

When all's said and done, high-carb day is a day to enjoy yourself. The recommendations I give in terms of quantities are not specific to the Pyramid Diet and, yes, of course they will vary from person to person. I want you to be able to make sensible, educated decisions yourself from the word go. Diets which begin by keeping you on a short rein, then gradually loosening it, are ultimately doing things the wrong way round. What's the good in restricting your intake of a certain food group, or cutting your calories substantially, then, once you become thinner and your body needs less fuel to sustain your weight, opening the floodgates again? It's totally irrational. Just because you've changed physically and *look* slimmer, does not mean to say you can resist those inevitable temptations. That is why the Pyramid Diet is the only diet with genuine life-time sustainability.

I hope you enjoy high-carb day and that you use your net-carb limit wisely. Now it's time for me to introduce you to Day 2.

8. Day 2: Low-Carb Day

Hopefully you will find that Day 2, low-carb day, follows on from the high-carb day nicely. On the low-carb day, you will not be able to have so many carbs, but you'll still be allowed up to 0.5g per lb of body weight. There are diets out there that are 'low-carb' and will not allow you to eat anywhere near as many carbs as this. (Remember, tomorrow you will have a day of no carbs, so don't kid yourself there is no discipline required.)

Based on the assumption, once again, that you weigh 140lbs, you can have up to 70g of carbs on the low-carb day. (And again, you will be working with net carbs, so make sure you deduct the fibre from the total carb figure.)

A Typical Low-Carb Day

	Net Carbs
Meal 1: Fruit and fibre yoghurt pot	16g
Meal 2: ½ cup cottage cheese and fresh fruit	20g
Meal 3: Tuna and egg salad	0g
Meal 4: 30g cashew nuts	5g
Meal 5: Chicken breast with cajun sweet potato (large), broccoli and spinach	25g
Meal 6: Almond butter cookies	4g
Total	**70g**

As on the high-carb day, you are not on a mission to consume your full net-carb allowance. It is simply in place to ensure you do not exceed your limit. If you weigh 140lbs and only consume 60g of net carbs on the low-carb day, that is fine. It's always better to come in under your allowance than creep over.

Moderating your carb intake to keep it at a reasonably low level can be a challenge at first. Many standard-sized meals could just tip you over the limit depending on your body weight. A 185g serving of lentil curry with 100g brown rice would provide around 50g of net carbs. For someone with a carb limit of 70g on low-carb day, this is entering dangerous territory.

In my experience, it is more satisfying and mentally rewarding to distribute your carb allowance relatively evenly throughout the day. So this same person with the 70g allowance on 5 meals a day would be able to enjoy 14g net carbs per meal. Their diet could look something like this:

	Net Carbs
Meal 1: 2 slices granary toast with a 4 egg omelette	25g
Meal 2: Apple with low-fat cottage cheese	10g
Meal 3: Good-carb stir-fry with chicken	2g
Meal 4: Natural live Greek yoghurt	8g
Meal 5: Salmon fillet with green beans and cajun sweet potato	25g
Total	**70g**

At first glance, this doesn't appear to be low-carb at all, and I hope it goes to show you do not have to feel you are missing out or living on chicken and egg whites to keep within your boundaries. In fact, I challenge you to ask a friend what they make of the menu above. I'm confident they will deduce it is healthy, but I very much doubt they will guess it is low carb!

The Pyramid Diet assists you in making those tiny tweaks towards bringing your net-carb intake down just a notch or two. That is one of the things that makes this diet so exciting and surprising. Choose the *right* carbs with a high amount of dietary fibre, combine them with protein-based foods to lower the GL and, bingo, you will have everyone around you baffled as to how you are losing weight whilst still eating 'normally'.

Eating Out

Eating out on a low-carb day follows the same principles as a high-carb day, so if you are having your evening meal in a restaurant, you'll probably find you'll eat many of the same foods you would have done on the high-carb day. So long as you stay within your weight limit, feel free to enjoy fresh fruit and wholegrain products when available.

Protein

Try to make sure you are getting 1g of protein per lb of body-weight. As always, you will find the tables in Chapter 16 useful to calculate your daily intake.

Why You Need the Low-Carb Day

I've often been asked what the point of low-carb day is. At first glance, it comes across as the middleman who doesn't really do much except stand in the way of getting the job done. In order to trick your body and dip in and out of anabolism and catabolism, surely you only need alternate between high-carb and no-carb days, right?

To a certain extent, this is correct; however there are several good reasons for slotting the low-carb day in between the two extremes:

- Day 2 allows for enjoyment without over-indulgence. Adding a low-carb day into the mix every third day makes for fewer high-carb days, whilst still allowing you to enjoy a limited amount of carbohydrate foods.
- Low-carb day does not totally deplete your glycogen stores, yet it keeps your total food intake down in line with your daily energy requirement.
- Day 2 is the best day for exercise (see below for more details)
- Once you have reached your desired weight, you may wish to bend the rules a little from time to time. While it is not advisable to have two consecutive high-carb days, it is acceptable to have up to three low-carb days in a row. We will speak more about this when we discuss 'The Pyramid for Life' in Chapter 12.

Exercise

Low-carb days are the most flexible days for exercise. They are the only days on which you are advised to perform both cardiovascular (aerobic) and resistance (weight-bearing) exercise. They allow for fat-burning as your glycogen levels are not too high; however, you will also have sufficient glycogen stores to do weight-bearing exercise too. If you're a gym bunny, take advantage of this and have a nice long workout on Day 2.

Small Errors Add Up

Whilst the above demonstrates low-carb day is not terribly restrictive, there are some pitfalls that are all too easy to fall into, especially where drinks are concerned. A 250ml serving of skimmed milk contains 11g of net carbs and these all add up when you're drinking it in tea and coffee throughout the day. If you're partial to the odd latte, you'll need to be even more careful. Fluids often get overlooked where diets are concerned, but calories in carbs, protein and fats all go down the same hole, regardless of whether you sip or chew!

Twenty-one-year-old hairdresser Hollie Burkett found this out when she began indulging in milky coffees through-out the day at work.

'I was drinking between five and ten hot drinks a day, with two sugars and way too much milk. Because it was fluid, not solid food, it didn't really occur to me this would cause me to gain weight. When I saw a picture of myself as a bridesmaid in a figure-hugging dress, I was shocked at how much weight I'd piled on in just a few short weeks. Aged just 19, I'd gone from a super-slender size 8 to a size 14, seemingly overnight. My clothes were very tight, but looking back I was in denial and carried on squeez-ing into them anyway. When I was forced to shop three dress sizes larger than I was used to, I decided to contact Danni.

HOLLIE'S STORY

'We sat down and scrutinized my diet; took it apart and put it back together again. Danni explained that whilst it was most likely the sugary, milky drinks causing the weight-gain, I was going to have to change the way I ate if I wanted to regain

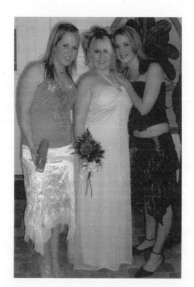

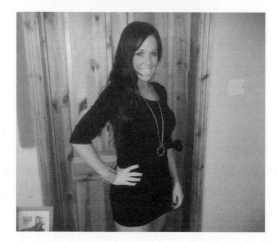

(top, left) Hollie as a bridesmaid
(bottom) The revived size 8 Hollie

my former figure. I wasn't used to eating breakfast, or lunch for that matter, but I soon got used to it. To be honest, what is there to complain about if you're told you need to eat *more* food to lose weight?!

'I'm no Gordon Ramsay but I learned the basics of cooking because I accepted I wasn't going to lose weight by living on toast. Buying fresh food has been great, because I've actually found I save money and have more left over to spend on things like holidays.

'The only things I've really cut out of my life are the sugary drinks. I can still have takeaways, which is a life-saver on a Friday night after a busy week at work, and I can still enjoy wine in moderation, which I also have a slight penchant for.

'It took me three months to get back down to a size 8 and I learned a valuable lesson along the way: Sugar makes you fat! The Pyramid suits me perfectly and I've even introduced a few of the girls at work to it. Now that I own my body again, I am never going to let it slip away!'

Don't Go Too Low!

Low-carb day is just as much a part of the jigsaw puzzle as the high-carb and no-carb days. As we'll see in the next chapter, no-carb day is pretty straightforward, in that you have an upper-carb limit of 20g regardless of your body-weight. High-carb day allows 1g net carbs per lb, and whilst you are not required to hit this figure, most of you will because your body will be craving carbohydrates by the time this day comes around.

That leaves us with low-carb day. Although there is an upper net-carb limit in place, you are by no means obliged to hit it. But go too low, and you will simply be re-living no-carb day. It is essential you do not do this, as the Pyramid is a three-day cycle and as I have clearly stated before it is not intended to be a purely catabolic or no-carb regime. Low-carb day has been put in place for a reason and I want you to sensibly enjoy carbohydrates on this day.

9. Day 3: No-Carb Day

If the idea of having no carbs makes your palms sweat, please relax. You will find your body adapts to the high-, low-, no-carb cycle naturally and will crave fats and proteins on Day 3, so you should find it relatively easy to cut out stodgy carbs such as bread, rice, pasta and potato every third day.

You're not expected to be a dietary nun, and for this reason you have an allowance of 20g of net carbs on no-carb day (excluding green fibrous vegetables, which are unlimited). This allowance comes irrespective of body-weight for ease of calculation. Use it as an approximation but don't exceed this figure, regardless of whether you weigh 150lbs or 300lbs.

Whilst you are never encouraged to be anti-carb on the Pyramid Diet, Day 3 is all about cutting them out, just as Day 1 is all about piling them up. Cheat just a tiny bit and you won't keep your body guessing. Remember, the Pyramid is a three-day cycle that needs to be staggered to work effectively. Having a high-carb day followed by two low-carb days will not achieve the same effect as cutting out carbs entirely on Day 3.

Because you won't be consuming calories from carbohydrates, you will need to increase your intake of fats and proteins. Wondering how to do this? All of the foods below contain 5g or less of net carbs in a typical serving, and most provide a decent amount of protein and/or fat.

- Fish: Salmon, tuna, sardines, mackerel, cod, trout, prawns, swordfish

— Meat and poultry: Chicken, turkey, beef, lamb, pork
— Animal/dairy products: Eggs, low-fat cheddar, cottage cheese
— Nuts (with the exception of chestnuts)
— Fruits: 1 small orange, 1 kiwi fruit, ½ grapefruit, handful of berries, 1 small plum, 1 small apricot
— Yoghurt: 80g of Greek yoghurt or natural, live yoghurt
— Good-Carb Steam Fry (see p232)
— Fibrous green vegetables (the darker green the better)
— Olives

A Typical No-Carb Day

So what does a typical no-carb day look like? You'll recall that on high-carb and low-carb day I based the sample menus on an individual weighing 140lbs. No-carb day differs in that everyone has an upper net-carb limit of 20g regardless of body-weight. Therefore, the following menu is suited to all Pyramid followers.

	Net Carbs
Meal 1: 4-egg-white omelette with mushrooms and spinach	0g
Meal 2: Smoked salmon-stuffed Avocados (p224)	2g
Meal 3: Chicken and vegetable stir-fry (eg, mushrooms, pak choi and broccoli)	5g
Meal 4: Cottage cheese with celery to dip	0g
Meal 5: Grilled tiger prawns	0g
Meal 6: Cod Steaks with Garlic and Saffron Aioli (p232)	2g
Total	9g

Eating this menu would use only 9g of your 20g net-carb quota for the day, but it is important to stress that on no-carb day the 20g limit is an absolute upper limit. Any carbs you do consume should ideally come from vegetables, so putting this allowance towards starchy carbs such as bread and pasta is wholly unadvisable. And if you drink tea or coffee with milk, you will need to take this into consideration. An average hot drink with a splash of skimmed milk will give you around 1g of net carbs. Many of us can get through 5–6 cups of tea or coffee a day, so that's an extra 5–6g! The Pyramid Diet is forgiving, yes, but it will not be effective unless you keep to the cycle, and blowing your net-carb allowance on no-carb day is probably the most damaging thing you can do to your waistline.

Eating Out

If you have a meal out scheduled on a no-carb day, what is the best way to tackle it? Believe it or not, there are a variety of dishes you can still eat with friends or colleagues without making it obvious you're on a diet. Here is an example of a no-carb three-course meal at a variety of restaurants with a total net-carb count of under 10g:

Italian

- Starter: Tiger prawns or scallops
- Main: Salmon and green vegetables or chicken in a red-wine sauce
- Dessert: Strawberries or raspberries (no sugar)

Avoid pasta, pizza, rice, potato, garlic bread, chips and sweet desserts.

Chinese

— Starter: Plain spare ribs or chicken satay or clear chicken soup
— Main: Beef, chicken or fish with soy sauce or black-bean sauce and steamed veg
— Dessert: Lychees (small portion)

Avoid rice, noodles, sweet and sour sauce, plum sauce, pancakes, spring rolls, barbeque sauce, battered chicken or pork balls, sweet desserts.

Indian/Thai

— Starter: Chicken tikka kebab (no sauce)
— Main: Small Thai green curry (no rice) or small chicken tikka masala (no rice) with curried vegetables if desired
— Dessert: Small portion of fruit

Avoid Bombay potatoes, rice, chapati, naan bread, onion bhajis, samosas, thick curry sauces and sweet desserts.

It almost goes without saying that sugar is strictly prohibited on the no-carb day, as on any day whilst following the Pyramid Diet, but there are plenty of ways to satisfy a sweet tooth with fruit.

Twenty-four-year-old mum of two Gemma Timms learned the hard way when it came to suffering the effects of a high-sugar diet. As a busy mum, she'd snack on boiled sweets, then cook refined foods such as pizzas and chips at meal-times. Gemma was always skinny as a child and even lost her baby-weight relatively easily, but once she fell into the sugar trap, her slender figure became a thing of the past.

'Because I was always a super-skinny size 6, I was used to being able to eat whatever I wanted and not gain an ounce. After I had my children, the baby-weight seemed to disappear without too many problems and I remained skinny for a few months after my second child.

'When the children started eating solid foods, things became very hectic in the kitchen. I wasn't really sure how to cook, but I knew it was important for the kids to have green vegetables and three square meals a day. By the time I'd finished their dinner I was exhausted, so I'd just throw a pizza in the oven for myself or survive on a pack of sweets. I could eat a family-sized pizza in one sitting and at first I didn't really think about the implications.

'Looking back, I suppose before I had the kids I had a fairly well-balanced diet, because I used to visit my mum quite regularly for tea, and I didn't really touch pizza at all. I assumed I could abuse my body and get away with it; but I was wrong.

'When I weighed myself one day and found out I'd gone from 8 to 12 stone I was devastated. I didn't even weigh that much when I was pregnant! The worst part was, I knew now that I'd gained so much weight it was going to be tricky to lose it again and I'd have to find something sustainable that I could stick to.

GEMMA'S STORY

'Devoid of any cooking skills or nutritional knowledge, I considered trying a low-carb diet because I'd heard this was the quickest way to lose weight and change the way your body metabolizes fat. I tried this method for one day, but it was no good; the extremely high-carb and high-sugar lifestyle I'd been living meant I just craved sweets and pizza too much to keep it up. I caved in that evening and ordered myself a huge meat feast. I felt depressed, alone and ashamed that I'd let myself go so much. That was when I found out about the Pyramid method.

'When I first started the Pyramid Diet, the only thing I really missed was the boiled sweets. I buy wholemeal pizza bases and add my own toppings like low-fat cheese, chicken, mushrooms, onions and peppers at home, which is great for both myself and the kids. I switched to granary-seeded bread and brown pasta instead of white, and I banned fizzy drinks from the house. When I craved something sweet, I'd simply have a piece of fruit and the cravings soon went away. Within six months I was back to my former self again and I now wear a sensible (but not super-skinny) size 8. I feel as if I'm in the best shape of my life and I even had some glamorous photos done!

'Low-carb day did present a bit of a challenge at first, because I was so used to eating processed foods, but now I know how to knock up a vegetable stir-fry with chicken or beef and get to enjoy things like poached eggs with lean bacon for breakfast, I'm not complaining!

'The Pyramid Diet has not only benefited me, but the children too. I didn't realize it was so easy to cook healthy food that doesn't cost an arm and a leg. I'm so happy I managed to turn my life around before it was too late. Fad diets? No thanks! How many people can say they can eat pizza and still stay slim?'

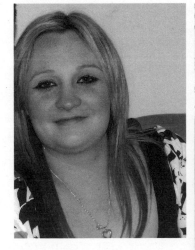 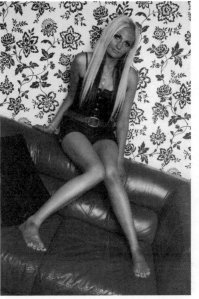

(left) Gemma weighing 12 stone
(right) Gemma now

Protein and Fat

No-carb day keeps your body's insulin levels low enough to allow for maximum fat-burning while retaining lean muscle. This is why it's really important to make sure you consume plenty of protein and fat on Day 3. To recap, you need to aim for at least 1g of protein per lb of body-weight. And when it comes to fats, don't just pile anything on your plate. Look back at Chapter 5 to remind yourself which are good and which are a no-no.

Fibre

Wholegrain foods such as brown bread provide a substantial amount of dietary fibre on Days 1 and 2, but of course they're not allowed on Day 3. Instead eat green fibrous vegetables in unlimited quantities. They are low calorie, filling and nutritious: 120g of broccoli contains just 29 calories, and the same amount of spinach on your plate comes in even cheaper, at just 24 calories. Remember, the darker green the vegetable, the more fibre it contains. Look back at the list on p49 or refer to the tables in Part Five to see which vegetables to avoid.

Salad is also a great way to fill your plate on Day 3, but be wary of tomatoes. One medium tomato contains around 2g of net carbs and they all add up. Opt for lettuce, radishes and cucumber, and coat with a good lashing of olive oil.

Beware of Potential Pitfalls

Sometimes, no matter how hard we *think* we are trying, there is still something standing in the way of sweet success. This is never truer than on no-carb day, where one innocent mistake could scupper the entire Pyramid formula. An example of this is milk in tea and coffee. Half a pint of skimmed milk contains around 13g of net carbs, so with a few milky cups of tea or coffee you could drink most of your carb allowance for the entire day.

Cast your mind back to Chapter 5, when I told you the way in which the juicing process strips fruit of its essential fibres, making fruit juice a bad choice for anyone wanting to stay slim. If you find yourself developing a sweet tooth on no-carb day and you're tempted to reach for the juice, think again!

There's no better person to vouch for this than 33-year-old Fiona Lee from Sandwich. I met Fiona on the set of *Bigger Than . . .* when she was competing to become a Katy Perry lookalike.

Fiona joined the show feeling fat, frumpy and out of shape. She didn't do any exercise and says she used to snack on 'all the wrong foods at all the wrong times'. Prior to applying, she started drinking orange juice in the belief it was doing her body good by contributing to her five-a-day and stopping her snacking on too many sweets.

At the first weigh-in, Fiona was a size 20 and tipped the scales at 16st 9lbs. Her waist measured a whopping 45 inches. She broke down in tears and made a promise to herself she'd never gain a single ounce of fat again. Fiona not only embraced the dietary challenge, she also made a vow to engage in physical exercise, and boy did she deliver – just four weeks after she first started training, Fiona successfully swam the Channel!

When we looked at what she had been eating and drinking, it was clearly the orange juice that was causing her to pile on the pounds. There wasn't all that much junk food in Fiona's diet, but as someone who was susceptible to putting on weight and already displaying the warning signs of insulin resistance, Fiona needed to realize that fruit juice was just as damaging to her body as some of the junk she'd managed to stay away from. Fiona cut the juice from her diet and replaced it with water and tea with a small amount of skimmed milk. During training, Miguel and I allowed her to consume a few extra carbs on no-carb day because she was exercising to extremes in the cold.

However, she still managed to follow the Pyramid Diet very well and the results spoke for themselves.

Fiona says: 'I never realized just how much damage all the orange juice was doing! I wouldn't have dreamed that drinking fruit juices could lead to weight-gain. I thought that only happened with fizzy drinks. As soon as I cut out the juice and hit the exercise hard, I managed to make positive changes to my body. Very positive, in fact. I've managed to stick to the Pyramid Diet since leaving the show and have continued to get slimmer and slimmer. Danni calls me the "shrinking lady", which makes me feel fantastic!'

Fiona lost a total of 2st 3lbs in 8 weeks, dropping from 16st 9lbs to 14st 6lbs. Her waist went from 45 inches to 36. She now wears a dress size 16, and says she hasn't finished losing weight yet.

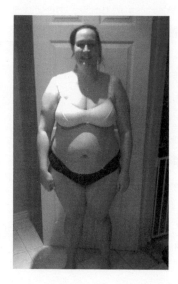 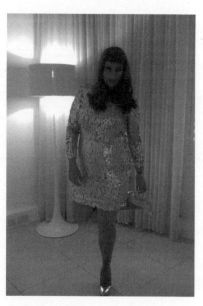

(left) Fiona at size 20
(right) Proud size 16 Fiona

Exercise

Because your body will be in fat-burning mode, you are encouraged to make the most of no-carb day. Remember, your body's insulin levels will be low, which will allow for some super fat-burning, so why not take a swim or go for a long brisk walk? For those of you who prefer to exercise in a group, try something like a spin class at the gym.

10. The Pyramid for Vegetarians and Vegans

This chapter is for any of the increasing numbers of vegetarians and vegans in the UK who want to experience the wonderful benefits of the Pyramid lifestyle. Is it possible to make the Pyramid work for you as well as for a carnivore? You bet!

As a vegetarian or vegan, you may feel a little overlooked by modern diet trends, with most low-carb diets placing a lot of emphasis on eating meat. An integral part of the Pyramid Plan is ensuring you recognize and appreciate the importance of protein from all sources. Hopefully you will already be aware of many of the vegetarian and vegan options and include plenty of these in your daily diet.

Some Veggie Vices

I am not saying this applies to every veggie on the planet, but there is one vice many veggies fall foul of. While meat-eaters tend to eat too much low-quality, fatty meat such as fast-food burgers and hot dogs, veggies often load their plates with starchy carbs like bread, pasta and rice. Because these foods are supposedly low in fat, I've come across many veggies (and indeed meat-eaters) who are under the impression this is a more healthy way to live. You now know the real devil is refined carbs, and if you're a pizza- or pasta-loving veggie, this evil substance may have total control of your dietary life.

In my mind, these refined carbs are just like a drug. We become addicted to them and our bodies feel as if they 'need' their next fix. It's not until we go cold turkey that we realize how much damage they were doing. Just be on your guard, because veggies are often fed this sort of thing in hotels and restaurants. But I think that if you choose not to eat meat, you deserve a meal rich in lean protein just as much as meat-eaters, so don't accept the cheap rubbish when dining out, and don't buy it either!

Yes, it's going to be harder for you to sieve out these foods than it will be for the meat-eaters, because they have probably formed the basis of many of your regular meals. There will still be an opportunity to enjoy wholegrain carbs, of course, so cutting out the damaging processed types will be easier than you think as soon as your body adapts.

I have divided this chapter into three sections. Just select the part that applies to you, then implement my instructions along with all the usual Pyramid guidelines.

Pescetarians

If you eat fish and seafood, things are very straightforward in terms of adapting the Pyramid to your own dietary requirements. Some of you may well be ahead of me and already enjoying your new way of life. If you're one of them, well done! You may still find it useful to make a few notes though, as you never stop learning.

Fish can offer a fantastic source of protein and omega-3. It also boasts the added benefit of being low in saturated fat. You can compare and contrast the protein contents of various types of fish and seafood in Chapter 16.

There are of course certain forms of fishy foods to avoid. I may be in danger of stating the obvious here, but under no circumstances should you be consuming 'convenience' seafood such as fish fingers, cod or haddock in batter, crabsticks, frozen fish in butter sauce, or fish-made-into-appealing-shapes and then frozen. You need not be a culinary sensation to learn to grill a piece of salmon, or bake a fillet of cod with fresh tomatoes and olives. Begin by experimenting with some of the simple recipes in Chapter 15, or pick up one of the free booklets that are available at the fish counter of most supermarkets.

Most of us enjoy fish as a starter or as a main course for lunch or dinner. However, there are many ways in which to enjoy fish and seafood throughout the day, so open your mind to these opportunities.

- Granary toast with poached kippers and brown-rice vinegar makes a wonderful breakfast.
- Smoked salmon on cucumber or raw courgette slices is ideal as a snack.
- Cottage cheese and anchovies on endives is a delicious protein-packed snack or light lunch.
- Try sardines on granary toast with cracked black pepper for an omega-3-filled lunch.
- Cod's roe on thin granary toast makes a decadent appetizer or canapé.

Vegetarians

If you're a vegetarian (i.e. you don't eat fish and seafood but do eat eggs and dairy products), the possibilities are still endless. You are probably already accustomed to foods such as Quorn in your daily diet, but if you're a meat-eater looking here for interesting and cheap sources of protein, you might like to know a bit more about this fantastic product.

Mycoprotein: The Pyramid-Approved Alternative

Quorn is made from mycoprotein, a member of the fungi family, naturally low in calories and high in fibre. It contains no cholesterol, all the essential amino acids found in meat, is lower in fat than beef and tastes delicious too. If you are not vegetarian, there's no reason why you can't still incorporate mycoprotein into your diet.

Aside from these health perks, mycoprotein may well be a powerful tool in reducing blood-sugar levels and bringing the all-important glycaemic load of meals down. A study in 1995 concluded that the insulin response in all of the subjects was lower after consuming a mycoprotein meal than it was after a 'control' meal.* The only nutritional difference between the two meals was the higher fibre content of the mycoprotein meal, which contained 11.2g more fibre. This not only outlines the importance of dietary fibre to you yet again, but means that mycoprotein is an excellent choice for the Pyramid Diet.

If you're already eating Quorn in your diet, let's spice

---

* 'Mycoprotein reduces glycemia and insulinemia when taken with an oral-glucose-tolerance test', Turnbull and Ward, *American Journal of Clinical Nutrition*, vol. 61, 1995.

things up a little. You'll find a range of delicious recipes online that show there is more to mycoprotein than ready-made sausages or burgers. However, the same rules apply when cooking with Quorn as they do with animal protein. Meals that include carbohydrates such as rice and pasta must only be consumed on high- and low-carb days and within the upper-carb limits in place for that particular day. And of course refined white carbs are out. The positive impact of mycoprotein on blood-sugar levels will be compromised or negated if you ignore these rules.

Why Eggs Are Everything They're Cracked Up to Be

If you're a vegetarian who enjoys eggs, you may nevertheless be a little confused by the great egg debate. Some say they're the best thing since sliced bread, offering an excellent, safe source of protein, others that egg yolks are high in cholesterol and therefore should be consumed with caution. Shall we settle this once and for all? Here's what Miguel Toribio-Mateas has to say:

MIGUEL SAYS ...

'We need eggs. They are a great source of protein and the trace element sulphur, necessary for the production of the hormone thyroxine (produced by the thyroid). Unless you have high triglycerides and/or liver-function problems, it is perfectly fine to have up to 8 eggs per week. In addition, it is safe to eat as many egg whites as you like. For example, I normally advise making omelettes with 4 whites and 1 yolk to get the balance right. Always try to use free-range eggs, which are naturally more nutritious.'

Eggs are delicious poached, fried with extra-virgin olive oil spray, scrambled with skimmed milk, boiled, or used to make omelettes. Include some chopped mushrooms, spring onion, olives and tomatoes in your omelettes for a scrumptious breakfast, lunch or dinner. Slice a boiled egg to form part of a protein-packed tuna salad, or even top tuna or swordfish with a poached egg to impress guests. Quail's eggs are great for this purpose, as they are smaller and more delicate than hen's eggs.

Dairy Proteins

Don't be tempted to overdo your dairy intake as a way of supplementing your protein intake. Whilst these products are a perfectly credible source of protein, they also tend to be high in saturated fat and pose a high intolerance risk. We discussed lactose intolerance at some length in Chapter 5, and if this is something you suffer from it is imperative you steer clear of milk and cheese. Yoghurt with live bacteria is OK, as you have already learned, but if you must drink milk, the only options are soya milk or milk with the lactase enzyme added.

Other dairy products have a more impressive amino acid–carbohydrate ratio, and these can make some super veggie snacks. Cottage cheese, which we have already spoken about, fares much better than full-fat Cheddar cheese and is delicious eaten at any time of day. Natural, live Greek yoghurt can also make a fantastic breakfast, lunch or snack when eaten alone or accompanied by fresh fruit.

Vegans

If you're a vegan, you've already struck quite a few devilish foods off the list. The process by which ready-meals are made, even Quorn products, means you will not be buying packaged foods, and the vast majority of junk food is banished too.

All that's left for me to discuss are the strongest forms of protein from which you can get your 1g per lb of body-weight per day. The following is also relevant to all Pyramid dieters.

MIGUEL SAYS ...

'Beans are a fantastic source of protein. The best in my opinion are split peas, lentils and chickpeas. Nuts and seeds are also great, with almonds and hemp seeds topping the chart, followed by cashews and many others. Being vegan does not mean you have to miss out on the Pyramid RDA of 1g of protein per lb of body-weight. The only thing you'll really be missing out on is the saturated fat found in some cheap animal meats.'

Nuts and seeds make fabulous snacks, whilst split peas, lentils and chickpeas can form the foundations of delicious soups, curries and other hearty, nutritious dishes. They are cheaper to buy than meat or fish and a little really does go a long way. Have a look at Chapter 15 to find some vegetarian Pyramid recipes containing beans and nuts that are easily adapted for vegans. Canned beans are fine, but, as always, do not buy those containing added sugars. Alternatively, buy the beans dry and soak them overnight before cooking.

The Veggie Verdict

- Do not replace meat with refined carbohydrates; instead opt for an alternative source of protein.
- There are plenty of fish in the sea, so don't be afraid to explore the fabulous variety of flavours it has to offer.
- Mycoprotein comes with the Pyramid seal of approval.
- We benefit from eggs, so don't cross them off your list.
- The amount of protein in milk and cheese is overrated. Consume only in moderation.
- Beans, seeds and nuts are wonderful sources of protein for everybody, not just veggies.

PART FOUR

Making the Pyramid Work for You

11. Know Your Body

No matter how well a diet plan or fitness programme is formulated, there are some individuals who need slight adaptations – for instance, because of a medical condition that prevents them from eating certain foods, or requires them to eat things that would not normally be allowed.

Making alterations to the plan is something that should only be done if entirely necessary. There is a fine line between medical requirement and neuroticism. We've all made excuses for things during our lifetimes, and losing weight (or rather failing to!) is probably one of them. I will keep this chapter brief, but I hope that by the end of it you will be sensible and honest enough to differentiate between fact and wishful thinking.

So that you can be sure the Pyramid is safe for you to follow, below is a list of common medical and dietary conditions, along with advice on any alterations that are possible. You should consult your GP before starting any new diet plan if you suffer from any of the conditions below, or any condition that may pose similar dangers.

Diabetes

Diabetics will need to alter the Pyramid in accordance with their own condition. However, on the whole, you should find that the low- and no-carb days will actually help to alleviate your symptoms thanks to the low GI/GL of all approved food items or food combinations.

Miguel Toribio-Mateas advises Type I and Type II diabetics to remove high-carb days entirely and alternate between low- and no-carb days:

'The insulin-resistance characteristics of diabetes means that your body can't react to high levels of blood sugar, so high-carb day is a no-no, as it will send your sugar levels rocketing. However, all other elements of the Pyramid plan should work well for you, so just alternate low- and no-carb days, forming a two-day cycle instead of three.

'All Pyramid-approved foods and food combinations are low GI and low GL, so anything marked 'approved' in the tables passes the diabetic checkpoint. If in doubt, always include a source of protein (meat, fish, dairy, eggs or pulses) with your carbs to minimize a detrimental impact on your blood-sugar levels. If you feel unwell, please stop the diet and contact your GP or diabetic nurse immediately.'

Before we move on, I just want to take this opportunity to discuss diabetes in more detail. This condition is on the increase in Britain. Children as young as *eight* are now developing Type II diabetes, which twenty or thirty years ago was only seen in people over fifty. In my opinion, childhood is the most important time in our nutritional lives; it is when we develop likes and dislikes, dietary habits and a psychological approach to food. If you are a parent, you have a duty to protect your children from the dangers of diabetes and to educate them about the risks associated with it. This will enable them to continue a low-risk diet once they are old enough to make their own food choices.

In order to lessen your family's chances of developing Type II diabetes, make sure you cut down on refined carbohydrates, sugar and alcohol. The Pyramid Diet helps you to make these choices without even realizing it, but why not pass these changes on to your children too? You can never instil dietary sense too early. Don't induce eating disorders by causing them to fear fatty or sugary foods, but make silent moves towards a better lifestyle on their behalf. Strip the cupboards of bleached carbohydrates and sweets and replace these foods with wholegrains and natural sugars found in fruits. Make sure food is a friend, not a foe, for your children, and give them a real chance of avoiding the dietary yo-yo when they grow up.

Nut Allergies

The Pyramid Diet places quite a large emphasis on nuts as a credible source of dietary protein and versatile ingredient, but if you suffer from a nut allergy I'm sure you realize that it is imperative that you are not tempted to incorporate nuts into your diet for any reason.

Lactose Intolerance

We discussed lactose intolerance at length in Chapter 5, but if you think you may suffer from this condition, you should get tested. This is a service most doctors' surgeries provide if you are experiencing discomfort after consuming dairy products. If you prefer, there are also a wide number of private food-allergy clinics around the UK. For a fee, these clinics will test your body's responses to a variety of foods and normally give you the results on the same day. This is something well worth doing if you suffer from bloating, IBS or digestive problems.

Wheat Intolerance and Allergies

Wheat intolerance is yet another common ailment that often goes undiagnosed. Symptoms include fatigue, bloating, diarrhoea and constipation. It is often misdiagnosed as IBS or chronic fatigue, leaving sufferers helpless and uncomfortable. The term is in many ways misleading, as in fact there are three main types of wheat 'intolerance' that vary widely in severity. Understanding which condition you suffer from is essential for formulating a suitable diet.

Wheat Intolerance

A wheat intolerance should not be confused with an allergy. Whilst an intolerance can cause discomfort, the symptoms of bloating, diarrhoea, etc., are not usually as violent or acute as those resulting from an allergy. The sufferer may not experience symptoms for hours or even days after wheat ingestion, and consequently, wheat intolerance can be difficult to diagnose. If you believe you may suffer from a wheat intolerance, there are investigative routes available. If in doubt, it is a good idea to avoid wheat or consume only very small quantities, which may allow you to build up tolerance.

Celiac (or Coeliac) Disease

Celiac Disease is an allergic response in the intestinal tract to a protein called gliadin. This is a gluten protein contained in wheat and several other grains, and consequently celiac disease is often referred to as a 'gluten allergy' or 'gluten intolerance'. If left undiagnosed and the sufferer continues to eat foods containing gluten, damage can be done to the intestinal tract. The good news is that the treatment is simply to follow a gluten-free diet, and many suitable food products are now widely available.

Celiac is a life-long condition, which cannot be cured. If you think you may suffer from it, don't leave it any longer to get tested, because much of the damage done to the body can be repaired once you remove gluten from your diet.

Wheat Allergy

The term 'wheat allergy' also refers to an allergic response to wheat, but in a broader capacity. Whereas celiac sufferers react poorly to gliadin, someone with a wheat allergy may have a reaction to many different proteins found in wheat and related cereals. A wheat allergy can be gastrointestinal, but it can also act in a similar way to hay fever, inducing asthma-like symptoms such as a runny nose and a cough, as well as hives, rashes, contact dermatitis and itchy eyes.

A wheat allergy can be extremely dangerous, sometimes even life-threatening. As with celiac, avoidance of wheat is the prevention, but the condition cannot be cured. If you suffer from a wheat allergy it may be the case that you are able to tolerate alternative gluten-containing grains, such as barley and rye, but this really is specific to the individual and is something that should be professionally assessed by your GP or an allergy clinic.

Underactive Thyroid Gland

An underactive thyroid has to be one of the most popular excuses in the dietary bible. The condition is not that common, but nowadays you can almost guarantee that if your friend, mother or family pet is overweight, it's their thyroid causing the problem. It's almost like diagnosing yourself with asthma as an excuse not to go running!

Not been tested but still convinced you suffer from an underactive thyroid gland? Possible, but unlikely – in the UK only around 15 in 1,000 women and 1 in 1,000 men suffer from the condition.* If you are overweight, have tried every trick in the book, stuck to a clean diet over a reasonable period of time, exercise regularly but still cannot seem to shift the bulge, there is a chance you may be one of them. In this case, visit your GP, who will give you a definitive answer.

High Cholesterol

If you've been diagnosed with high cholesterol by your GP and prescribed medication, you need to be extra vigilant about consuming fatty foods and try to cut saturated fats out of your diet. Typical low-carb diets may well not be suitable for you, as they do not discourage the consumption of fatty meats and full-fat dairy products such as whole milk and

* All figures from www.nhs.uk

cream. Following the Pyramid Diet will help you cut these damaging fats out of your life.

Food labelling can be confusing, but if you suffer from high cholesterol, it is saturated fat you need to be aware of, as this affects your cholesterol levels more than eating high-cholesterol foods themselves. The NHS website states: 'If your GP has advised you to change your diet to reduce your blood cholesterol, the most important thing to do is cut down on saturated fat. It's also a good idea to increase your intake of fruit, vegetables and fibre.'

The Pyramid Diet will help you along with this nicely, whether you suffer from high cholesterol or not. The only Pyramid-approved foods you should consult your GP about are whole eggs (specifically egg yolks) and prawns, which are higher in dietary cholesterol than most foods. However, the chances are your doctor will give you the go-ahead to eat these in moderation, because, as I pointed out above, the cholesterol found in food affects your own cholesterol levels far less than the amount of saturated fat that you eat.

Irritable Bowel Syndrome (IBS)

IBS is a common condition affecting millions of people world-wide. It is one of the most common digestive conditions, affecting an estimated 10–20 per cent of people at some point in their lives.

If you are one of these people, you will be familiar with the discomfort caused by bouts of bloating, stomach cramps, diarrhoea and constipation. There is no cure for this irritating condition, but you can relieve your symptoms by altering your diet and lifestyle.

IBS is not a dangerous condition, and whilst it is uncomfortable, it poses no serious threat to your health. If you suffer from IBS on a very regular basis (weeks or months can pass between flare-ups in some people), there are medications available. Discuss this with your GP and avoid trigger foods, which often appear to cause your symptoms to escalate.

This chapter is called 'Know Your Body' for a reason. You may be familiar with all the conditions listed above, but the fact remains that many of us simply do not suffer from them; the sooner we accept that being overweight is usually the result of over-eating and lack of exercise, the better.

I meet so many people who are overweight – and indeed many who are within the normal weight-range – who are adamant they suffer from a medical condition that prevents them either from exercising or from making the right food choices. But those who have fabricated or 'assumed' these ailments are only cheating themselves.

To follow the Pyramid Diet effectively, you need to be both responsible and honest with yourself. The diet encourages you to get to know your own body and listen to what it is telling you. It does this in a number of ways:

- By not dictating that you count calories or restrict your total food intake.
- By making you aware of common allergies, ailments and medical problems, and informing you of the necessary steps to diagnose and alleviate these conditions.
- By encouraging you to engage in physical exercise to enhance weight-loss and complement the positive medical effects of the Pyramid Diet.

- By letting *you* decide when you have reached a weight you are comfortable with, and setting your permanent net-carb limits accordingly.
- By allowing you to consume alcohol in moderation and at your own discretion, but not to the detriment of your health or weight-loss.
- By giving you the freedom to adapt the Pyramid Diet to suit your lifestyle and deviate from the set pattern accordingly. This is something we will discuss in greater detail in the next chapter.

Ultimately, no one knows your own body better than you, and it will be you setting your limits for carbs, fats, calories and alcohol. Do not under any circumstances make excuses for deviating from Pyramid rules, unless medically advised to do so.

The same goes for exercise. If you suffer from asthma, high or low blood pressure, bone, muscle or joint problems, arthritis or back pain, there may be limits to what you can and can't do. However, once again, the onus is on *you* to know your own body and listen to its needs. If you have a dodgy knee and it genuinely tells you not to walk any farther, stop walking. But if you have a dodgy knee and your GP has told you it is safe to walk, yes, you might get bored after 10 minutes, but *keep walking for at least 30 minutes*! Quite often, your mind will tell you what you *want* to hear, when in fact you just don't fancy the exercise! (Remember too that many exercise-induced aches and pains are simply from joints having to bear too much weight. This should only tell you one thing; you need to be doing *more* exercise!)

If you get bored easily when working out, try setting yourself a fitness challenge or training with a friend. Exercise does not have to mean running on the treadmill for hours. If you are fortunate enough to pursue an active hobby, such as tennis or horse riding, make the most of this and invest as much spare time into getting physical as you can. I have witnessed physical activity cure numerous clients of depression, as well as helping them to lose weight. I cannot emphasize the benefits of exercise enough, and I hope that you embrace this as a fundamental part of the Pyramid programme.

We are now about to move on to 'The Pyramid for Life', and explore the ways in which you may adapt the Pyramid to suit your lifestyle long-term. If you give in to temptation easily, I ask that you do not read the next chapter until you have reached your desired weight through the basic Pyramid structure, as you may be too tempted to stray from the yellow brick road.

12. The Pyramid for Life

I've no doubt that for many of you, this is the chapter you've been looking forward to most. I hope that in some cases, you've re-opened this book having reached your goal weight and are now ready to move on and apply the Pyramid principles to the rest of your life. If you are choosing to read this chapter before losing the desired amount of weight, please do not be tempted to implement anything too flexible too soon unless medically necessary. Remember, the only person you are cheating if you do this is yourself.

Lose Weight and Keep It Off

Way back in Chapter 2, we talked about some of the flaws in popular modern diets, and I explained how the Pyramid formula keeps you away from the dreaded yo-yo.

I seldom meet a person who cannot lose weight, yet the majority of people struggle to keep it off. A few short months, weeks or even days after reaching our target weight, we wake up to find those excess pounds we fought so hard to shed have begun creeping back. We ask ourselves what we've done wrong, and why we are plagued with the 'fat gene' when we've gone to such efforts. But no one gives us the answers, and no one comes to take the unwanted fat back. And so, disappointed as usual, we resign ourselves to that 'one pizza' or 'single takeaway' and the cycle resumes.

If this rings bells for you, you are not alone. Being over-weight requires more than a temporary solution, so how can a short-term or quick-fix diet possibly offer long-term relief? It can't. Losing weight is not just a physical process; it's a state of mind. If your mind is in the right place, your eating patterns will follow.

Changing Habits for Life

Unfortunately, where eating and drinking are concerned, we may be in charge of the controls, but we don't listen when our brains tell us certain foods are no good, or our bodies tell us we're full up, or we've had too much to drink. And some-times, the more intense the binges, the more inclined we are to repeatedly turn the gun on ourselves. Eating is a very pleasurable experience. Over-eating is not. It makes us feel uncomfortable and often unwell, leading to physical symp-toms and ill health. So why do we do it to ourselves?

There is very often a psychological explanation for weight-gain and I want you to try to identify this in your own mind. Stress, relationships, depression and lack of self-confidence are all well-documented reasons for letting our figures slide. Everybody wants to take control of their lives, and over-eating, like under-eating, is a form of control, a channel through which to express power, frustration, guilt, happiness or shame.

Clearly if you think you have serious problems with under- or over-eating, you should go to see your doctor, but most of us should be successful in breaking our damaging eating habits after just a few weeks on the Pyramid Diet. Because it is a plan for life, it will never leave you feeling you've come to the end. Sure, you can loosen the belt a little from time to time, but remember, a diet is not a 'journey', it is a way of life.

Change, Not Restriction

The relationship you have with your body is not just physical. It's our brains that tell us what food and drink to put in our mouths, not our hands. And our brains decide whether we should walk or drive, sit or stand, take the escalator or the stairs. We are all creatures of habit and we all want to make life easy for ourselves, so we usually take the easy option. That is unless we make a conscious effort to change. At first, any change is difficult – and you should try to take it one day at a time – but as you get into your new Pyramid habits and your brain is gradually retrained, it will become easier.

There are two components of change associated with the Pyramid Diet. The first is the periodic reduction in net-carb intake until the desired body-weight is reached and a constant net-carb limit is set. The second is the constant change dictated by the pattern of the three-day cycle. The body needs change to burn fat. Ironically, if we want to maintain a constant weight, the most effective way to achieve this is by implementing constant change.

Another important aspect of Pyramid are the daily limits. We keep to plenty of these in other areas of life: the number of hours we can stay awake without nodding off, for instance, or the amount of cash we can withdraw from our bank. So we know we can do it, and I really hope that you feel guided by the limits set by the Pyramid Diet, not confined by them. Remember, it is outside of the Pyramid that is the real prison cell. Stay within the limits and you will experience more dietary freedom than ever before, particularly psychologically.

'There is nothing more imprisoning than yo-yo dieting,' says Miguel Toribio-Mateas. 'Sadly, not many people manage to break free of it once they get themselves in this dreadful downward spiral. Fortunately, the Pyramid Diet offers a solution.'

Tricks of the Trade

I am often asked for 'tricks' one can implement when craving sweet, sugary foods or processed snacks. I'm afraid there is no magic wand, and there are no secret crisps that are made from lettuce. One client recently asked me for a list of foods that he could eat as much as he liked. I had to break the news that, other than perhaps cucumber and celery, these foods do not exist.

It can be frustrating to have to accept that junk food is fattening. But in the vast majority of cases, I find that being allowed to eat the odd takeaway will suffice for most people. Cutting out processed, packaged food really is a small price to pay for a slender body you get to keep!

Make a list of your top five Pyramid-approved snacks and make sure you have them to hand both at home and in the workplace. That way, if you ever find yourself feeling peckish and tempted to nibble at something naughty, you'll be able to prevent yourself by exchanging it for a low GI, zero sugar, figure-friendly snack that tastes every bit as good.

The Golden Rule for Sustainable Weight-Loss

The Pyramid is for life, but life is never perfect. Realistically, you will not always keep to the perfect triangle. But as long as you stick to this golden rule, your new weight will be sustainable:

Never Indulge in Two Consecutive High-Carb Days!

Sound unfair? Let me show you something. The Pyramid Diet I laid out to you in the beginning went like this over a seven-day period:

— Monday: High-carb day
— Tuesday: Low-carb day
— Wednesday: No-carb day
— Thursday: High-carb day
— Friday: Low-carb day
— Saturday: No-carb day
— Sunday: High-carb day

The Pyramid Diet depends on an unsettled metabolic pathway, further stimulated by a low starchy carb intake, and there is no way to have back-to-back high-carb days whilst still reaping the benefits of the Pyramid cycle.

We all have different levels of self-control, and it may well be some of us are not in danger of breaking the nutritional boundaries on a high-carb day, but for the purposes of generalization I have chosen to implement this golden rule for the greater good of all Pyramid followers. Absorb it and respect it, or else don't embark on the Pyramid Diet.

The Forgiving Triangle

The Pyramid does have lifetime flexibility, which can be a godsend in certain social situations. Supposing you have a professional meal to attend one evening, followed by a friend's birthday dinner the next. What are you supposed to do if the restaurant menus simply do not offer carb-free options and you've just hit the no-carb day of your cycle? Relax; it's easy.

> If you have already reached your desired weight, simply replace the no-carb day with another low-carb day, then follow with a high-carb day as normal.

> If you are still trying to lose weight, count the celebration as a low-carb day, then insert an extra no-carb day, then carry on as normal to a high-carb day.

Of course there are numerous other circumstances that might crop up. Below I'll try to answer the most common questions about the flexibility of the Pyramid below.

FAQs

Q. What is the maximum number of low-carb days I can have in a row?

A. For the purposes of keeping your body guessing, you should not have more than three consecutive low-carb days at any time. However, *if* you reached your desired weight more than 3 months ago and you're 100 per cent comfortable with your weight, you may have two or three low-carb days, followed by a high-carb day, then return to a low-carb day.

Q. I want to speed up my weight-loss; is it OK to add in some extra no-carb days?

A. Absolutely not. For starters, it will not be conducive to permanent weight-loss. Secondly, the Pyramid Diet was not developed to encourage you to join the queue of people resorting to temporary anti-carb solutions. You will only shoot yourself in the foot and end up back on the dreaded dietary yo-yo.

Q. Do I absolutely have to include no-carb days in my diet?

A. As a matter of fact, no you don't. However, if you do, your new body will be much easier to maintain. Once you have reached your desired weight, the no-carb day is simply there to keep you in check. Think of it as being like your mother who reminds you to eat your greens when you visit for Sunday roast! Have a no-carb day every third day and you can rest assured your new body is safe.

Q. Do I need to exercise in order to lose weight?

A. No, but it certainly helps – a lot! This is discussed at length in the next chapter.

Q. If I deviate from the Pyramid Diet while on holiday and eat something like pizza, what should I do?

A. Whilst I do not encourage these choices, there is no point in kicking yourself when you're down. If, for whatever reason, you really can't stick to the plan whilst you're away, re-familiarize yourself with the Pyramid principles when you return from holiday and start again, being careful to follow the default three-day cycle for at least 30 days. You will soon start to appreciate the return to a more healthy way of life.

Q. Can I increase my upper net-carb limit for high-carb day once I have lost the desired amount of weight?

A. This is a very difficult question to answer, because some people can get away with it and others can't. If you are tempted to increase your carb limit, the weight can start to creep back on if you overdo it, and who's to say exactly how much your body can cope with? This is, in my view, a flaw of modern low-carb diets that allow you to work out your body's metabolic capabilities for yourself. Very often, you think you're maintaining the weight-loss, but in reality the fat is slowly but surely sliming its way back on to your hips and thighs.

Therefore I recommend that you stick to the simple and safe upper-carb limit of 1g per lb of body-weight. If you do choose to increase it, do this only on special occasions and immediately follow with a low-carb day to bring your system back into check.

The Water of Life

There is one more element of the programme that is so important, you must not ignore it:

You Must Drink a Minimum of 8 Glasses of Water a Day!

We covered the reasons why this is so important way back in Chapter 1, but it bears repeating here: if you allow yourself to become dehydrated, your body's fat-burning abilities are greatly reduced.

The Pyramid for the Journey

I could sit here and tell you what you want to hear, or I could exaggerate by telling you there is no room for error when it comes to the Pyramid. As you'll already have gathered, the truth is somewhere between the two. If you allow yourself a handful of crisps every day or a couple of slices of white toast every other day, you are more likely to regain weight than somebody who swears by Pyramid principles all week, then enjoys a large pizza and chips on a Saturday night. Don't get too excited, I'm not suggesting you binge to these extremes, but there is room for a 'cheat meal' every once in a while *once you have reached your desired weight*!

'Cheat meal' is a term commonly used by body-builders to describe a meal (usually once a week) of foods they wouldn't normally eat whilst dieting. This can be anything from a little gravy on their chicken to a huge burger and chips. Some say it helps kick-start their metabolisms, thus preventing that catabolic slow-down caused by prolonged periods of dieting. They also say that, psychologically, a cheat meal perks them up and helps to keep them going through the mental torture of strict pre-competition dieting.

The Problem with Cheating

If, once you've achieved your goal weight, a cheat meal is something you decide to incorporate into your lifestyle, I won't stop you from doing so once a week. However, I want you to be aware of the potential problems associated with loosening the belt, because for some people, just one cheat meal can be their first step back towards the dietary yo-yo.

The Pyramid is forgiving enough in itself, if you ask me — you can eat bread, you can eat pasta, and you can eat tasty desserts and fruit. If that's not enough and you want to cheat once a week then go ahead; but proceed with caution!

Possible repercussions of cheat meals include:

- Increased insulin levels. This decreases fat mobilization and oxidation.
- Potential problems with self-discipline for the hours and days following the cheat meal.
- Increased storage of fat around the body. It has been estimated that in the average person, consuming a meal consisting of over 750 calories leads to measurable fat storage. This is regardless of the macronutrient content of the meal and purely based on calorie content. The only exception to this rule is consuming a high-calorie meal in the post-exercise window, which we will discuss in the next chapter.
- An increased percentage of energy comes from carbohydrate oxidation, while a decreased percentage of energy comes from fat oxidation.
- In my view, the negative effects of consuming a cheat meal outweigh the positive effects of 'stoking the fire' or shocking your metabolism. Remember, the Pyramid Diet is already designed to keep your body guessing on a day-to-day basis, whilst maintaining a safe level of control.

The Verdict

If I were you, I'd avoid cheating, but once you've reached your desired weight, feel free to play around with the Pyramid structure as described above. It's your life, it's your body and it's your Pyramid, so make it work for *you*!

One Pyramid dieter who's made it work for her is 37-year-old Georgina Upcott from West Sussex. Georgina was almost 19 stone before starting the diet, and now weighs 15st 3lbs. She's gone from a size 24 to a size 18 and says she still wants to lose more weight, but decided to adapt the Pyramid to her lifestyle once she reached a size 18.

Georgina says: 'Unlike a lot of people who go on diets, my goal was never to be a size 8. I enjoy being curvy, but I did feel as if I was too overweight at almost 19 stone. I didn't want to enrol on some fad diet, because I enjoy good food and I didn't have a specific time-frame in mind for losing the weight, so long as I 'got there'. I also wanted a plan that I could adapt to suit my own lifestyle that didn't make ridiculous demands on my wallet, or require me to eat according to the colour of my front door!

'The Pyramid plan has worked perfectly for me, because I lost the weight without even thinking about it and have now reached a high-street size 18. Now that I've achieved this, I would like to take things a little further and get to a size 14–16, but I'm in no hurry. I decided to throw an extra low-carb day in here and there, because whilst I am still losing weight, I did reach my initial goal and I know I will continue to slim down so long as I adhere to Pyramid guidelines.

'My diet was not all that bad before, but making simple changes such as cutting out sugar and switching to wholegrains seems to have helped my metabolism, which has always been slow. I'd recommend the Pyramid to anyone who enjoys their food. Why give up your favourite meals when you don't have to?'

GEORGINA'S STORY

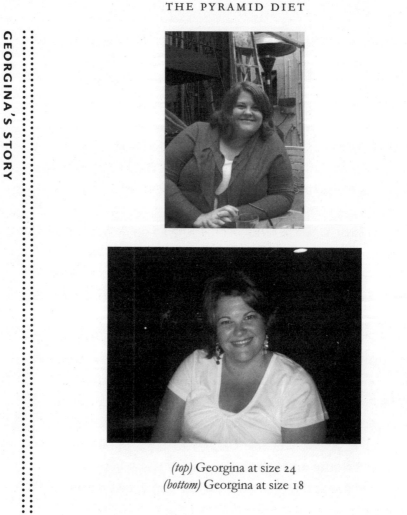

(top) Georgina at size 24
(bottom) Georgina at size 18

13. Why Exercise Matters

Dozens of well-known faces claim to hold the key to slender success. But if you've tried all those fitness DVDs and feel like giving up, try one more thing before you do, because I believe it's the only thing guaranteed to stop the endless yo-yo journey you've been on.

Look at the science – and I'm not talking white coats and microscopes, but plain and simple facts. None of these diet and exercise gurus attempt to educate you as to how your body actually works. And when it comes to shifting those excess pounds and achieving the body shape you desire, how can you succeed if you don't understand why you're doing what you're doing?

In this chapter I'm going to explain to you how many muscles in the body work, why certain movements work certain areas and which types of exercise are best suited to which days on the Pyramid Diet. Your body is an engine; without fuel it would grind to a halt, but put the wrong fuel in and you're in for a bumpy ride – in more ways than one!

First things first; there are a few home truths I need to get off my chest. I am confident that at least one of the questions below concerns you. The information I am about to give you is the truth, the whole truth and nothing but the truth, so please accept the facts and take them on board!

Do I Have to Exercise to Lose Weight?

No, you do not *have* to exercise to lose weight. If that's all you wanted to know and you are certain you are never going to move a muscle, I won't argue with you. But please read a bit further before you skip to Chapter 15 and enjoy yourself in the kitchen instead. Still with me? Fantastic! I am now going to take you through some of the ways in which physical activity can enhance and speed up fat-loss.

Exercise and Your Metabolism

In Chapter 2 we spoke about how the Pyramid Diet helps to speed up your metabolism and stops it from grinding to a catabolic halt. But wouldn't it be great if you could give it an even bigger boost and turn it into a lean, mean, fat-burning machine? The good news is, you can. Everybody can teach their bodies to stop storing fat and start burning it.

The bottom line is that if we eat more food than we need, a certain amount of it is going to be stored as fat around the body. And it's not just the fat you can see that you need to worry about, but also the fat you can't.

INVISIBLE FAT

You'll recall how excess carbohydrate (glucose) is converted into glycogen. It is then stored around the body as subcutaneous fat, visceral (abdominal) fat or deep down, out of sight, in the muscles or liver. Too much subcutaneous fat and we become visually unattractive and overweight, with damaging physical and psychological consequences. Too much visceral fat was thought for a long time to directly affect our risk of developing insulin resistance, diabetes and cardiovascular disease. But in 2009, scientists at Washington University School of Medicine discovered that in fact it is fat deposited in our livers that has the strongest link with the development of these diseases.*

We all eat slightly more than we should at times, so how can we minimize the problem? By now it will probably come as no surprise to you that a healthy diet coupled with regular physical activity is the *only* way to eradicate both the visible and invisible fat. Cast your mind back to Chapter 2, when we spoke about the metabolism and the ways in which the Pyramid Diet sparks off a tug of war between anabolism and catabolism, keeping your body guessing and increasing the speed at which your metabolism works for you. We are now going to take this one step further.

YOUR METABOLIC RATE

Your basal metabolic rate (BMR) is the number of calories the body burns at rest. You can view your BMR as the total amount of calories you'd expend if you remained in bed asleep all day. In the average person, this accounts for about 65–70 per cent of their total metabolism. So what makes up the remaining 30–35 per cent? Well, we use between 5 and 10 per cent digesting and absorbing food, then about 7 per cent for the body to produce heat to regulate our temperature. The remaining 13–23 per cent goes towards – you guessed it! – physical activity.

* 'Intrahepatic fat, not visceral fat, is linked with metabolic complications of obesity', Fabbrini, Magkos *et al.*, *Proceedings of the National Academy of Sciences*, vol. 106, 35, 2009.

The percentage of total metabolism consumed by physical activity varies from person to person depending on how active they are. We all know that exercise helps you to lose weight by burning calories. The great news is that it can do more than this. Exercise helps to raise your BMR by building lean muscle tissue, which is more metabolically demanding than fat tissue. This means that someone who exercises will burn more calories at rest (even when sleeping) than a sedentary person.

Of course there are other factors that go some way towards determining your BMR, but many of these are fixed things you cannot influence, such as age, genetics and gender. The amount of physical activity you engage in is something you *can* change, so give yourself the best possible chance of boosting your BMR and improving your body shape by engaging in something that gets you moving.

If I Build Muscle, Won't I Put On Weight?

As you have probably heard a thousand times, muscle weighs more than fat. But there is something else you need to know (and once you know it, it is glaringly obvious): *muscle has far greater density than fat*. It's like that trick question about which weighs more, 1lb of feathers or 1lb of lead. The fact is that 5lb of muscle simply takes up a lot less space than 5lb of fat. So if you gain 5lbs of fat, the surface area will be larger, lumpier and more unattractive than if you gain 5lbs of lean muscle.

Not only does lean muscle help you to burn fat, thus reducing your overall body-weight and size, someone weighing 150lbs with 20 per cent body fat will appear slimmer and lighter than someone of the same weight with 35 per cent fat – even though technically they weigh the same.

We concern ourselves far too much with weight, as opposed to body composition. A simple body-fat test can help you to determine roughly what percentage of your body is fat. A more complex test carried out by a professional clinic will be able to determine this more accurately, and will take visceral fat into consideration. As I've said before, always use a dress size, waist size or favourite pair of jeans as a goal, not body-weight.

If I Lift Weights, Won't I End Up Looking Like a Body-Builder?*

I know that many of you believe that if you lift weights you'll turn into a muscle machine. This is simply not the case; there are dozens of different ways to perform weight-bearing exercises to help you improve your body shape and fitness levels, no matter what your age, sex or body type.

This is generally something that concerns women to a greater degree than men. Often when I've asked a woman to pick up a weight for the first time, I can immediately see I've put the fear of God into her. But as somebody who regularly works with athletes who grace the world of female muscle, I can tell you they did not achieve that look by throwing a

* There will be a minority of you reading this book as the first step to building visible muscle. Carb-cycling is a great way to achieve this, but the Pyramid Diet is geared towards those simply wanting to lose fat and develop a lean, toned figure. For a hypertrophic diet, for which you will need to increase both your carbohydrate and protein intake, please refer to specialist body-building literature.

3kg dumb-bell around! The image of a female body-builder you probably have in your mind right now is something that requires an enormous amount of hard work, dedication and *heavy* lifting. Not only that, women don't produce enough testosterone naturally to achieve those muscles, so a lot of these women take synthetic testosterone, as well as other supplements. Without hours spent lifting very heavy weights and taking these supplements, there is no way on earth you are going to look like a female body-builder.

I hope that I've cleared up these questions for you once and for all, and that you can share this knowledge amongst friends and loved ones who, for whatever reason, were refraining from exercise.

The Different Types of Exercise

Moving swiftly on to the exciting stuff! Perhaps you've already started the Pyramid and are seeing changes already. If so, give yourself a huge pat on the back. For those of you who've not yet embarked on the diet, now is the time to get cracking! And no matter what stage you're at, there's no better time than the present to get moving.

You may have tried diets that dictate you must not engage in vigorous exercise until you are past the introductory phase – that is, the initial phase of starvation or food-group deprivation where your body is so depleted, it cannot safely perform the movements and functions it is designed for. This should have been enough to make you close the book there and then! On the Pyramid Diet, it is safe to do any type of exercise right from the start. If you are new to working out, or you've not exercised for a few years, take your time and start slowly. You'll soon begin to see and feel the benefits and will be able to progress at your own pace.

There are two types of exercise that I'm going to talk about: cardiovascular and resistance, and it is imperative you understand the benefits both types have to offer.

Cardiovascular Exercise

Cardiovascular, or 'cardio', exercise normally refers to aerobic exercise. (It's not *always* aerobic, but you don't need to concern yourself with the scientific nitty-gritty for now.) Aerobic exercise can be anything from walking to running, playing tennis to cycling, swimming to rowing, and is all about getting your heart rate up. Some of the numerous benefits of aerobic exercise include:

— Burning body-fat
— Increasing lean muscle tone (toning up)
— Improving circulation and reducing blood pressure
— Reducing the risk of diabetes
— Strengthening muscles throughout the body
— Reducing stress

Resistance Exercise

Resistance exercise refers to the types of exercise that require some form of resistance to force the muscle to contract. This can be provided by anything from a dumb-bell to your own body-weight. It not only helps to improve body shape, but also bone health. And as you'll remember from our discussion on basal metabolic rates, because muscle tissue is metabolically active, the more of it you have the more calories you will burn, even at rest.

These are just a handful of reasons why I believe weight-bearing exercise of this kind is hugely underrated in a woman's world.

Which Should You Do?

Some say cardio is overrated, whilst others argue it is the only form of physical activity necessary for developing a shapely body and burning fat. The verdict? There are no short cuts and in order to reap the maximum benefits, you need to be doing both. We'll go into more detail later in this chapter, but before that I'd like to introduce you to Megan, a twenty-two-year-old financial advisor.

MEGAN'S STORY

At 12st 2lbs and size 16, Megan felt fat, frumpy and out of shape.

'I'd always tell myself I was happy being overweight, but I wasn't. I used to kid myself when I looked in the mirror and tell myself I was slim, but I knew sooner or later I'd have to face the reality that I'd be better off if I were a few pounds lighter. I wasn't dangerously overweight, just chubby, and I think that made things harder to accept. I'd dipped in and out of various diets and been a member of the gym, but without any real structure things always seemed to fall away after a couple of weeks and I'd go back into a state of denial.

'That all changed when one day I was looking at pictures of myself in a bikini on holiday with my parents. We'd just got back to the UK and I'd dashed out to process the photos right away. When I saw myself in print, I was horrified. I looked far bigger than I thought I was! It was time to face the music. I started training with Danni four times a week and have followed the Pyramid Diet religiously ever since.

'I've managed to lose 2st 2lbs and now weigh a healthy 10st. I've gone from a size 16 to a size 10 and have even done some modelling work. I feel beautiful, and now I can be confident in the knowledge I look beautiful too. Now, when I look in the mirror I always remind myself that what I see is what everyone else sees. It's no good kidding ourselves, because matters only get gradually worse as time goes on.

'Exercise is now a crucial part of everyday life, and is something I wouldn't give up for the world. I'm now so full of energy

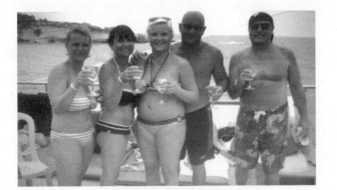

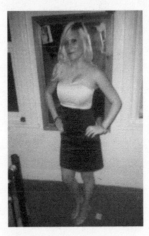

(top) The family holiday photograph that gave Megan a wake-up call.
(bottom) Megan enjoys dressing up for nights out now
that she's a perfect 10!

my friends and family can't keep up with me! I can't believe I lived the way I did for so long. I thought it was normal to feel tired and bloated all the time; now I know this is not the case. Without exercise I don't believe I'd have achieved such dramatic changes in my physical appearance or become so much happier and more confident in myself. I love running and always try to go before work on no-carb days, but resistance exercise is a lot of fun too and has given me a body shape I'd never dreamed of!

'The best thing about the Pyramid programme is the way in which the diet and exercise components complement one another. I love being told when to perform certain types of exercise as it gives me some structure. Without this, I don't think I'd ever have been able to succeed.'

What, When and How?

First I'd like to reassure you that it is perfectly safe to perform either cardiovascular or resistance exercise on any given day, regardless of whether it is high-, low- or no-carb. However, for best results, follow the Pyramid guide to exercise and let the two components of the programme work in harmony. Here's a quick recap of the best days to do each type of exercise.

High-Carb Day

Remember, the purpose of high-carb day is to fill your glycogen stores and stave off muscle catabolism. So high-carb days are the perfect time to give those muscles a good workout, and do resistance exercise to really tone up that body.

High-carb days are not ideal for doing a cardio activity such as cycling or running. This is because insulin inhibits fat-burning, and your pancreas will be secreting more insulin on this day than any other. If you're already an avid aerobic athlete and can't keep away from the treadmill, go ahead, but if you do take a day or two's rest from cardio, try to make sure it falls on high-carb day.

Low-Carb Day

Low-carb days are the most versatile of the three, ideal for doing both cardiovascular and resistance exercise. They allow for fat-burning as you will not be secreting huge amounts of insulin, yet at the same time your glycogen levels will not be too low to fuel a good old work-out with weights.

No-Carb Day

On no-carb days, your body's insulin levels will be low enough to allow for some super fat-burning. If you're a cardio king or queen, no-carb day is your time to shine. Make the most of your enhanced ability to melt fat on this day and find an aerobic activity that gets your heart pumping.

If you already engage in a physical activity you enjoy, the Pyramid Diet can help you make the most of your abilities in this area.

Meet 30-year-old Steve Gillespie. Before embarking on the Pyramid programme, Steve weighed 13st 12lb and had a waist circumference of 34 inches. He wasn't overweight for his height, nor was he unfit, but as a keen rugby player Steve decided it was time to up his game.

'The Pyramid Diet has helped me improve my speed and endurance through fat-loss. Not only that, I've improved on my PB [personal best] in all aspects of fitness. I've gone from 88kg [13st 12lb] to 81kg [12st 10lb] in seven weeks and my waist has decreased from 34 inches to 31. My body-fat percentage has also gone down from 22 per cent to 18. I'm really pleased, because I tried the Dukan diet and didn't notice any difference at all. Not only has the Pyramid Diet proved easy to follow, I've achieved things I always thought would take me far longer.'

What Time of Day is Best?

Making your exercise fit with the Pyramid plan day-to-day answers one component of the 'when'. But it does not address the most appropriate *time* of day.

In 2010 I came across a study in the *Journal of Physiology* that immediately caught my attention.* The experiment – which spanned six weeks and featured 28 healthy and active young men – was intended to test the effects of eating breakfast before exercise, eating breakfast and not exercising at all, and eating breakfast after exercise. All the while, the men were consuming a diet with a whopping 50 per cent more fat and 30 per cent more calories than they needed. Over this period, one would normally expect the subjects to gain weight. The findings were as follows:

Group A ate breakfast, then exercised. They gained an

---

* 'Training in the fasted state improves glucose tolerance during fat-rich diet', Van Proeven, Szlufcik *et al.*, *Journal of Physiology*, 588, 21, November 2010.

average of 3lbs over the six weeks and had started developing the warning signs of insulin resistance. They had also
begun to store fat within and between their muscle cells.

Group B ate breakfast and didn't exercise at all. Not surprisingly they packed on an average of more than 6lbs. They
had also developed insulin resistance and had begun storing
fat within and between their muscle cells.

Group C ate breakfast after exercise. They gained almost
no weight and showed no signs of insulin resistance, despite
following the same calorie- and fat-laden diet as the other
two groups. They also burned the fat they were eating more
efficiently than the other two groups.

The verdict: exercising in a fasted state (which is usually
only possible before breakfast) coaxes the body to burn a
greater percentage of fat for fuel, as opposed to relying pri-
marily on carbohydrates.

There is no magical explanation to this experiment. When
your body is depleted of glycogen, it calls on fat stores for
energy instead. Yes, one could argue that following a permanently carbohydrate-deficient diet and exercising at any
time of day would have the same effect. But letting your glycogen stores drop too low will have a huge impact on your
performance and really hinder your progress. The solution?
Carb-cycling, of course!

I hope by now you've learnt how important exercise is. By all
means exercise before breakfast if you possibly can, but generally speaking, the programme I'm going to give you in the
next chapter can be put into practice at any time of the day.
The most important thing is that you *do some exercise*! So read
on to start this vital part of the Pyramid programme.

14. Sculpt Your Body: The Pyramid 7-Day Exercise Programme

This chapter will give you an exercise programme to cover a 7-day cycle on the Pyramid Diet. In much the same way as I structured the diet, I have designed the training plan to be the best way to come out of the starting blocks. If further down the line you find yourself exceeding these physical demands or altering your exercise patterns, good for you!

Throughout the programme, I encourage you to work muscles that complement or assist each other on the same days. For example, the chest and tricep muscles are both activated when you perform pushing actions, so I've asked you to work them on the same day. This saves you both time and energy.

Before you begin: Always consult your doctor or physician before beginning any type of physical activity, and remember to warm-up and stretch before exercising. If you are new to exercise, it is a good idea to book an induction at the gym or a one-to-one session with a personal trainer to help get you started and check your technique.

The following movements are designed for both men and women of all ages and abilities. They can either be performed at home or in a gym if preferred.

Equipment for the Home

If you plan to do a lot of exercise in your home, there are a couple of pieces of equipment that you will need, all of which are readily available in high-street stores or online (e.g. www.dannifit.com).

A Swiss ball is a super piece of equipment to have and can be bought for less than a fiver. Be sure to buy the right size for your height: 55cm for 5'5" and under, 65cm for 5'6"–5'10" and 74cm for 5'11" and over.

A medicine ball is another great piece of equipment and comes in a variety of different weights. Start off with a fairly light ball and, as you get stronger, work your way up.

Day 1: High-Carb Day

Legs, Bum and Shoulders

Resistance exercise is a great way to tone up your legs and bum. Too many people mistakenly think running on the treadmill for hours and hours is the solution to orange-peel thighs and dimpled butt cheeks. They're wrong. The only way to effectively banish cellulite and get some shape to your legs is by targeting the muscles in these areas, namely the gluteus maximus (bum), quadriceps (front of thighs) and hamstrings (back of thighs).

Don't forget, weight-bearing exercise is great for improving muscle tone and faster fat-burning. The exercises below will see you on your way to shapely, sexy legs in no time!

THE PYRAMID 5-STAR EXERCISE: SQUATS

Target: Thighs and bum
Sets and repetitions: 3 × 12

Place your feet slightly wider than hip-width apart and pull your lower tummy in nice and tight as if you're sucking through a straw. Keeping your back straight, bend through the hips, then the knees into a nice deep-seated squat position. Squeeze your butt cheeks together as you straighten your legs to return to the start. Perform 3 sets of 12, taking 30–60 seconds' rest between sets. For extra resistance, perform this exercise with a bar-bell or dumb-bells. As an alternative in the gym, be brave and give the Smith Machine a go!

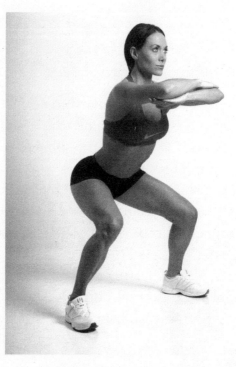

LUNGES

Targets: Thighs and bum
Sets and repetitions: 3 × 15 on each leg

Stand upright with your feet together. Fold your arms in front of you (as pictured) or, for added resistance, hold hand-weights down by your sides. Step forward with one foot, raising the heel of the back foot off the floor. Bend both knees until they are at approximate right angles. Push off the front foot to return to the start position. Repeat for 3 sets of 15 on each leg.

Handy hints: Ensure you do not lean forwards when performing the lunge. It is important to keep your torso upright

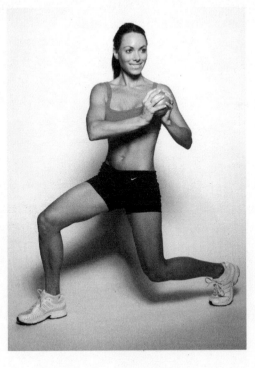

and your core muscles tight. Want to target your tummy too? Hold a medicine ball or hand-weighted object with two hands and twist your torso round to one side as you sink into the lunge (as pictured p197).

SWISS BALL HAMSTRING CURLS

Targets: Hamstrings and glutes (backs of thighs and bum)
Sets and repetitions: 3 × 15

Lie on the floor and place your feet on a Swiss ball with your arms by your sides, palms downwards. Lift your bum up off the floor high enough so that your body is in a rigid plank position. Keeping your core muscles tight for stability, slowly drag your heels in towards you, pulling the ball in as you do so. Keep your bum lifted throughout this process. Straighten your legs to return to the start position.

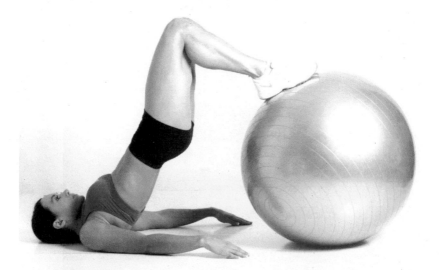

SWISS BALL BUTT LIFT

Targets: Glutes (bum)
Sets and repetitions: 3 × 20

Rest your upper back on a Swiss ball, then push your hips up towards the ceiling, squeezing your butt cheeks as you do so. Slowly lower your bum back down towards the floor. Repeat for 3 sets of 20.

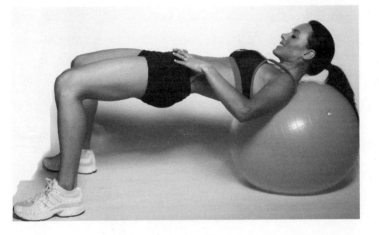

Handy hints: Losing your balance on the Swiss ball? Master this exercise by lying flat on the floor with your knees bent, before progressing on to the ball a few days or weeks down the line.

MEDICINE BALL HIGH THROW

Targets: Legs and shoulders
Sets and repetitions: 3 × 15

Holding a medicine ball up to your chest, bend your knees so that you are in a squat position. Keeping your chest up,

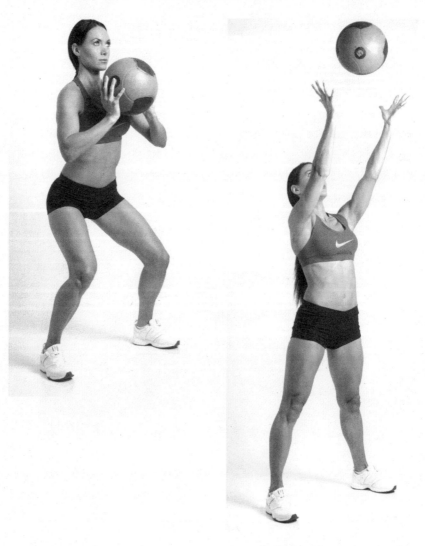

explode upwards, straightening your legs and pushing the ball up into the air as you do so. It is crucial that you fully extend the arms and really give the ball a good push in order to effectively work the shoulders. As you catch the ball, use its momentum to bring it into your chest, simultaneously sinking back into a squat position. Repeat for 3 sets of 15.

Handy hints: Start off by using a fairly light ball and, as your shoulders get stronger, work your way up. Toned shoulders will make your arms appear slimmer and more defined.

The Top Five Foods for an Anti-cellulite Workout

We can do all the exercise in the world, but if we want to avoid orange-peel thighs, complementing our fitness plan with an anti-cellulite diet is the only real secret to success. Here is my list of the top five foods that help to improve blood circulation, thus waging war on lumpy butts and thighs. These foods are all suitable for consumption on Day 1, high-carb day.

- Berries are particularly good at minimizing the appearance of cellulite, because they help combat free radicals, which attack cells, causing cellulite to appear worse. Try adding to sugar-free Greek yoghurt with live bacteria for a tasty breakfast.
- Asparagus is high in glutathione (GSH), an antioxidant that may help destroy cancer cells, and rutin, which is believed by some to strengthen veins, thus improving circulation. Better circulation means fewer lumps and bumps.
- Bananas are great for circulation and getting rid of toxins which congregate between the fat cells.
- Oily fish, rich in omega-3, helps our bodies to metabolize fats more efficiently and quickly.
- Nuts are a great source of essential fatty acids, which improve general health so that your body can get rid of the orange peel.

Day 2: Low-Carb Day

Cardio

Begin Day 2 with a medium-intensity cardio session lasting 30–60 minutes. For maximum fat-burning, do it before breakfast.

When I say medium-intensity, I want you to sweat, feel slightly breathless and have to give yourself an extra push to complete the last few minutes of the workout. I don't want you to feel totally exhausted, faint, dizzy or light-headed. For variety, why not try interval training, by fluctuating between inclines, intensity levels or speeds on gym-based cardio machines? This is a great way to increase your aerobic capacity and prevent boredom.

Acceptable forms of cardio include:

- Power walking (treadmill or outdoors). Add an incline or walk uphill to increase difficulty.
- Jogging or running (treadmill or outdoors)
- Cycling (gym bike or outdoors)
- Rowing machine
- Cross-trainer
- Stepper
- Spin classes
- Step or aerobics classes
- Swimming
- Zumba, salsa or other dance class
- Football, tennis, squash, rugby, hockey or netball

Resistance: Chest and Triceps

The tricep muscles, more commonly known as your 'bingo wings', are a tricky problem area for many of us. But with a combination of the right diet and a few simple exercises, you really can improve their appearance and start to feel confident in strappy tops or dresses.

PYRAMID 5-STAR EXERCISE: CLAP PUSH-UPS

Targets: Triceps (bingo wings)
Sets and repetitions: 3 × 5

Start off in a nice straight push-up position (see overleaf), ensuring you do not stick your bottom up in the air or let your hips droop down towards the floor. If you cannot manage this to begin with, do a half push-up by supporting yourself with your knees and crossing your feet over.

Keep your fingers pointing forwards and your hands beneath your shoulders. Lower your nose down towards the floor, then push upwards in an explosive movement. If you can manage it, clap your hands together in the air before landing back into a push-up. When you start out, you may only be able to take your hands off the floor for a split second. That's fine. Just make sure you don't let your weight transfer back on to your knees. You need to keep your weight forward and your shoulders over your hands.

Handy hints: Plyometric (explosive) exercises such as clap push-ups are great for the triceps and allow us to get some aerobic exercise in at the same time. The natural resistance offered by plyometric exercise also stimulates muscle growth, thus burning more fat and achieving a toned appearance. Rest between sets is very important, and the ratio of rest to workout should be 5:1, so I'd advise at least 30 seconds' rest after each set, during which time you can stretch.

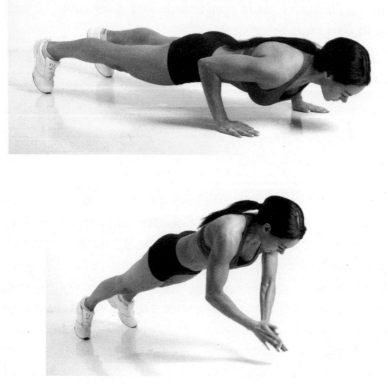

CHEST PRESS

Targets: Chest and triceps
Sets and repetitions: 3 × 12

Lie on a bench or a Swiss ball and ensure your head and neck are fully supported. Holding either a weighted bar or two dumb-bells in line with the centre of your chest, push the weight upwards towards the ceiling, extending your arms as you do so. Slowly bend your elbows to return to the start and repeat for 3 sets of 12.

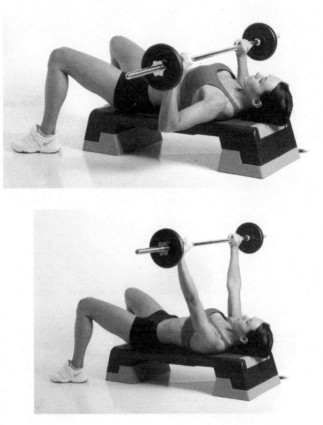

Handy hints: If you're female, the chances are you'll want to work on lifting your bust. An effective way to achieve this is by performing an incline chest press. For this, you need to work on a bench with an adjustable back rest. Lift the back rest until it is at a 45-degree angle. If you want to work your lower chest muscles, you'll need to do the opposite and lower the back rest so that you are sloping down towards the floor slightly.

SWISS BALL SEATED TRICEP EXTENSION

Targets: Triceps (bingo wings)
Sets and repetitions: 3 × 12 on each arm

Sit on your Swiss ball and make sure you have good posture
and your tummy muscles pulled in nice and tight (otherwise
you will miss out on the added benefit of working your core
muscles). Holding a dumb-bell, extend one arm up towards the
ceiling, supporting it with the other hand if desired. Keeping
your elbow pointing upwards as much as possible, lower your
hand down on to your upper back, bending your elbow as you
do so. Extend your hand back up towards the ceiling to contract the tricep muscle and repeat for 3 sets of 12 on each arm.

Handy hints: Moving the elbow out sideways is the most
common mistake when performing this exercise. It's really

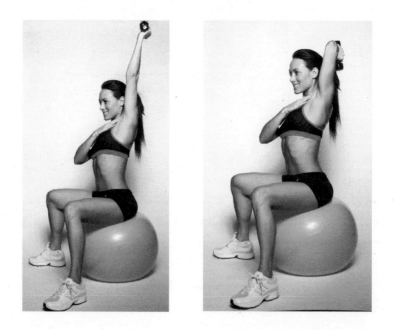

important that you keep the upper part of your arm still in order to isolate the tricep muscle.

Food For Thought

Ever ask yourself what foods cause excess fat on the upper arms? Well, the answer is just that: too much fat! Foods like chips and kebabs spell disaster. Not only do they contribute to cellulite and excess fat tissue, but also poor skin, which can often appear dry and patchy. A diet rich in lean meat, veg and the right carbs, on the other hand, will have you well on your way to beautifully lean triceps.

Other ways to improve their appearance are to reduce your salt intake – which will help reduce water retention – and to get plenty of omega oils, which will help improve circulation (and therefore cellulite) and dry skin.

Day 3: No-Carb Day

Cardio

No-carb day is the heavy-duty fat-burning day, and the best on which to focus on aerobic exercise. Remember the gorgeous Fiona from way back in Chapter 9? She owed a large percentage of her fat-loss to spending hours in the water, swimming her way to a slender body. Try to perform at least 45 minutes' cardiovascular exercise on no-carb day. If you are able to go one stage further and do a session in the morning (preferably before breakfast), then again in the evening, that would be ideal.

Day 4: High-Carb Day

Day 4 is your second high-carb day of the week. I don't want you to feel as if you have to exercise every single day. Rest is crucial to allow your body to make positive changes. For this reason, I am marking Day 4 as a 'rest day'. High-carb day is the best day to do this, as the insulin you will be releasing anyway inhibits fat-burning, so if there's one day I want you to sit back, relax and enjoy a wholewheat pasta dish, it's today!

Day 5: Low-Carb Day

Resistance: Tummy

Now is the time to introduce your tummy to a good workout. But before you begin, understand one thing:

> Unless you first get rid of the excess fat on your tummy, it will never look or feel firm, no matter how many sit-ups you do!

This is a really important point. In all my time as a trainer, it has been the most common misconception. Yes, exercise is important, but without the correct diet to strip the fat away, you are simply wasting your time performing hundreds of abdominal crunches. However, seeing as you're going to be following the Pyramid Diet so perfectly, I will now run you through the ins and outs of how best to train your tummy for a tight, toned, washboard torso.

Train Your TVA

Most people think about working their abs when they want to achieve a flat stomach. But there's a secret behind any wonderful washboard called the transverse abdominis (TVA), a flat sheet-like muscle that lies behind the rectus abdominis (the part we traditionally think of as our abs). The TVA is so vital to the appearance of our tummies that it has been nick-named 'the corset muscle'. Training your rectus abdominis alone will not give you a sculpted, flat stomach. It is merely the effects rectal abdominal exercises have on the TVA that lead the trainee to believe they are 'working their abs'.

The best exercise for the TVA is simply to sit up nice and straight in everyday life and contract the muscle by holding it in. Just imagine you're sucking up through a straw and don't allow your back to arch or your lower tummy to feel loose. If we can remember to do this, it makes an awful lot of difference when it comes to working out.

Want to go further to beat the bulging belly? Here's how:

SWISS BALL HAND-TO-FEET PASS

Targets: TVA
Sets and repetitions: 3 × 10

Lie on the floor and push down through your tummy button to ensure you are not arching your back. Stretch your arms up above your head. Grip the Swiss ball between your feet, then, keeping your legs straight, raise the ball up into the air, whilst simultaneously raising your arms up to take the ball from your feet. Pass the ball from your feet to your hands, then slowly lower your legs back down towards the floor at the same time as you lower your arms back down above your head with the ball. Reverse the movement, to pass the ball back to your feet and lower once again. Repeat for 3 sets of 10.

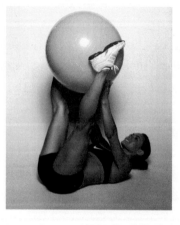

Handy hints: Don't have a Swiss ball? That's OK. You can perform this exercise at home using a football, cushion or anything you can easily grip your feet around. Just be careful you don't allow your back to arch, as this can cause damage to your spine and will negate the positive effects on the TVA.

If you have more time, perform some additional leg raises by lying on the floor with a flat back and slowly lifting and lowering your legs, keeping your arms by your sides. Once again, you should not allow for a gap between your lower back and the floor, and you must engage your tummy muscles before you start in order to prevent this.

The Six-Pack Muscles

In order to work a specific muscle, you need to shorten or contract it. For example, if you bend your knee you are working the hamstring muscle (at the back of the upper leg), because this part of your leg is getting shorter, and the front part is getting longer. Baffled? Try it now: Place your hand on the back of your thigh, halfway between your knee and your bum. Bend your leg a few times. Feel something working as you bend your knee? Excellent! Now let's apply this to the rectus abdominis – the second area of our tummies we should work on to improve the appearance of our midriffs.

SWISS BALL CRUNCH

Targets: Rectus abdominis
Sets and repetitions: 3 × 20

Lie on your Swiss ball and allow your head to flop back, creating a comfortable curve in your upper spine. Place your hands by your ears and keep your elbows pointing outwards. With your feet planted firmly on the floor, and your TVA engaged, slowly contract your tummy muscles to lift your head, shoulders and upper back off the ball. Keep looking forwards and slightly upwards, so that you maintain a constant gap between your chin and your chest. You should breathe out as you lift up, and in as you slowly lower back down to the start position. Repeat for 3 sets of 20.

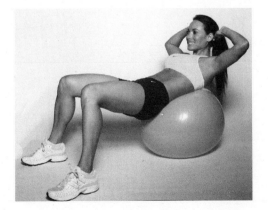

Handy hints: Struggling to stay on the ball? Practise this exercise on the floor first before progressing to the Swiss ball.

LYING TOE-TOUCH

Targets: Rectus abdominis
Sets and repetitions: 3 × 20

This exercise is great for those of you who are just starting out in physical activity, or who suffer from back problems. It can help you to regain your abdominal strength after childbirth, or simply help you to locate and establish the abilities of your tummy muscles when you first come out of the starting blocks.

Lie on the floor with your legs straight up in the air and your hands out-stretched towards your toes. Slowly lift your shoulders off the floor, breathing out as you do so, and slide your hands up your legs towards your toes. For added resistance, hold a medicine ball or similarly weighted object as illustrated. Perform 3 sets of 20 repetitions.

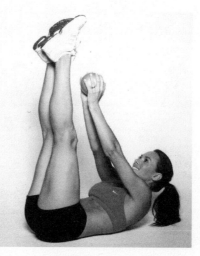

Handy hint: Do this exercise nice and slowly and it will really give your tummy muscles a thorough workout.

KNEELING PRAYER

Targets: Rectus abdominis
Sets and repetitions: 3 × 15

We work the rest of our bodies with weights, so why not our tummies? The 'kneeling prayer' shortens your abs whilst providing a gravitational pull for them to work against. You'll need to be a member of the gym to do this one, as it requires the use of a cable machine.

Kneel under the cable machine and take the ropes in both hands. With your TVA engaged and keeping your back straight, slowly lower your forehead towards the floor as far as is comfortable.

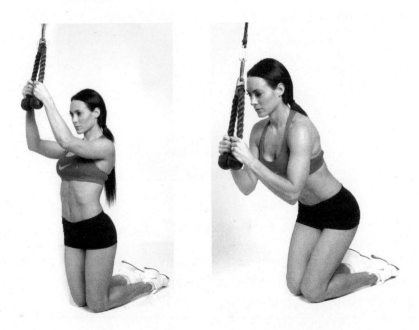

Handy hints: Keep the tension on your muscles and maximise the 'eccentric' (return) muscle load by making the return movement super-slow.

CRUNCH FROM FLOOR

Targets: Rectus abdominis
Sets and repetitions: 3 × 20

Lie on the floor with your hands by your ears and feet either flat on the floor with your knees bent, or in a raised position (as pictured). Lift your shoulders off the floor, breathing out as you do so, then slowly lower back to the start. Repeat for 3 sets of 20 and twist at the top of the movement if desired to hit the oblique muscles (sides of the tummy).

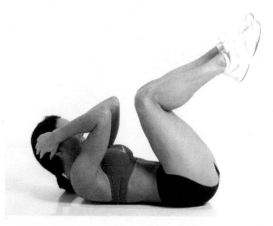

Cardio

Make use of your second low-carb day of the week by engaging in a good bout of cardiovascular activity, either before or after your resistance workout. Again, for best results do both before breakfast.

Day 6: No-Carb Day

Cardio

This is your second opportunity of the week to get moving in a *big* way, and burn maximum fat. So, again, try to do 30–60 minutes of your chosen cardio exercise, before breakfast if possible.

Day 7: High-Carb Day

Resistance: Back and Biceps

Day 7 is the final rung on the Pyramid exercise ladder, and is just as important as any one of the other six. The back and biceps are the only major muscle groups we have not yet addressed, and if you loathe the excess fat beneath your bra strap, don't neglect them! This is another exercise that you will need to do in a gym.

LAT PULL-DOWN

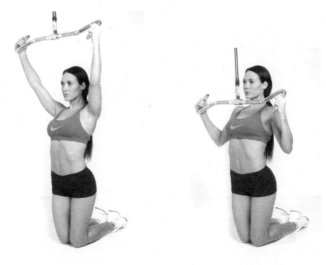

Targets: Back and biceps
Sets and repetitions: 3 × 12

This exercise can either be performed kneeling (as pictured) or seated on a fixed lat machine. Grip a lat pull-down bar so that your elbows are at approximate right angles when pulling it down towards your chin. Starting with your arms outstretched above you, slowly pull the bar down to just beneath your chin. Then, with precision and control, return it to the start. Keep your back straight and your tummy button pulled in nice and tight throughout.

PULL-UPS

Targets: Back and biceps
Sets and repetitions: 3 × 5

Most people avoid this exercise as it is thought of as 'hardcore' and only performed by body-builders and athletes. However, there are now a range of assisted chin-up machines available in all good gyms, which allow almost anyone to achieve this movement. I have chosen to include it in the Pyramid programme because for those of you who suffer from the dreaded 'bra strap fat', this is *the* exercise to banish it. Start practising it today, and reach for greater heights!

Simply hold the bar so that your upper arms are at right-angles to your body, and pull yourself up until your chin is above the bar.

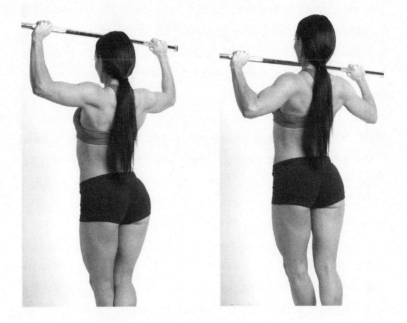

Cardio

It may be the last day of the week, but that's no excuse to neglect your aerobic duties. Keep it light, with a leisurely game of tennis, or a gentle swim. Whatever your chosen form of cardio, be sure to end the week on a high note!

Eating and Drinking for Exercise

I have dictated the exercise programme above to work in harmony with the Pyramid Diet. However, there are some additional factors you should take into account to enhance the positive effects exercise has to offer you.

Try to consume a lean source of protein within 90 minutes of exercise to help promote muscle repair and recovery.

The most appropriate (and least fattening) time to consume carbohydrates is actually just after exercise, when the body will be able to use them to replenish depleted glycogen stores. At this time, you will be less likely to store carbs as fat than at any other time.

Make sure you drink plenty of water before, throughout and after exercise to prevent dehydration and allow for optimum performance.

Don't fool yourself into thinking you 'deserve' to eat a kebab containing 600 calories because the treadmill tells you you've just burned 600 calories. Fat-loss simply doesn't work like that! If you're that intent on eating a kebab, forget the Pyramid Diet and go back to your old ways.

Sports energy bars and drinks often contain a lot of added sugar. Always check the label, and don't assume that just because something is available to buy in a healthfood store or from the gym vending machine, it is good for you. Most of the time these products will do you more harm than good.

Whilst I could preach the benefits of exercise to you until the end of time, I accept that both your time and interest are limited commodities. I truly hope you will make the decision to sculpt your body by incorporating physical activity into your lifestyle, and here I've given you the tools to do this within the Pyramid cycle.

I'm taking you on to the tasty world of recipes now, but please don't bury this chapter in the sand. It really will make a massive difference to what you can achieve.

PART FIVE

Recipes and Tables

15. Pyramid Recipes

Following the Pyramid Diet is far from boring for your taste buds, and in this chapter you'll see why. Whether you love Mediterranean flavours or savour a little spice in your life, you'll find plenty of delicious and easy recipes right here.

For those of you who are feeling adventurous, planning to hold a dinner party, or simply have a little time on your hands, I've included dishes to get you chopping, blending and baking your way to a healthier, more slender you. If you lead a hectic life and don't have the luxury of experimenting time, don't panic – there are a whole host of quick and simple suggestions for all three days on the Pyramid.

These recipes are unique to the Pyramid Diet and have been kindly donated by chefs and health experts from around the globe. I really enjoyed visiting such special restaurants and cafés, speaking to chefs and sampling these dishes, and I hope you enjoy making and eating them even more!

A few notes about ingredients: as a general rule, buy the best quality you can afford. Free-range meat is 'good enough', but use grass-fed whenever possible. And I'm sure by now you know that anything like tinned tomatoes or baked beans must have no added sugar. I've specified tinned pulses in most of the recipes, but of course you can also use dried, with the necessary soaking and cooking first.

I mention olive oil spray throughout. There are a few on the market, but the best in my opinion is FryLight's extra-virgin olive oil, which has added Vitamin E so that all the good omegas don't deteriorate at high temperatures. I also list soy lecithin, an emulsifier that thickens stews and sauces without needing flour. The granules can be bought at any health-food shop, as can the Vitamin C powder (a useful preservative), arame seaweed and Himalayan salt also listed. Himalayan salt is packed with minerals, but if you can't find it, sea salt is fine. Xylitol is a great sugar substitute for sweet dishes, and can be bought from health food stores and good supermarkets.

Each dish is labelled with its carb content and also the suggested day for consumption. So, for example, a dish containing 60g of net carbs could not be consumed on a no-carb day, but may be consumed on a high-carb day and possibly on a low-carb day (depending on your body-weight and the remainder of your daily diet). Just choose your dishes wisely when adding up the carbs, and don't be afraid to experiment.

Starters, Dips and Light Bites

HOME-MADE LIGHT MOROCCAN HUMMUS

The perfect snack any time of the day. If you're serving it to friends, surround the bowl with carrot and cucumber sticks, red pepper slices, chicory or endive leaves or any other raw vegetables.

Serves 3
Preparation time: 5 minutes
Cooking time: none
Total: 5 minutes
Suggested days: high- or low-carb
Net carbs per serving: 18g
Protein per serving: 9g

400g chickpeas, drained and rinsed
1 clove of garlic, peeled
30ml extra-virgin olive oil
2 tbsp tahini (unhulled if possible)
2 tbsp soy lecithin granules
juice of 1 lemon
1 tsp salt, or to taste
1 tsp ground cumin
1 tbsp goat's yoghurt
a pinch of Vitamin C powder (optional)
1 tsp smoked paprika (optional)

Put the chickpeas, garlic, oil, tahini, soy lecithin, lemon juice, salt and cumin into a processor and blitz to a knobbly purée.

Add the yoghurt and the Vitamin C powder if you're using it and process again. (The Vitamin C will make it last longer in the fridge.)

If the hummus is still very thick, add a little water. This will depend on the type of chickpeas you use. Taste for seasoning, adding more lemon juice and salt if you feel it needs it.

Sprinkle with the paprika if you wish, and serve.

Variations: add your own flavour with some blended raw red pepper, a little chilli, tomato purée, chicory or soft-boiled carrot.

SMOKED SALMON-STUFFED AVOCADOS

A versatile, flavourful meal. Makes an excellent brunch, a filling snack or a light supper.

Serves 4
Preparation time: 5 minutes
Cooking time: None
Total: 5 minutes
Suggested days: any
Net carbs per serving: 2g
Protein per serving: 5g

200g smoked salmon (wild or organic if possible)
2cm fresh ginger (or to taste)
1 spring onion
1 tsp lime juice
freshly ground black pepper
1 tsp tamari soy sauce
½ tsp balsamic vinegar

4 large avocados, peeled and halved, stones removed
2 tsp dried parsley
watercress to serve

Cut the smoked salmon into very thin strips and place in a medium-sized mixing bowl. Peel the fresh ginger and chop finely with the spring onion.

Mix the lime juice, black pepper, tamari sauce and balsamic vinegar in a bowl. Stirring vigorously, pour over the salmon. Add the chopped ginger and spring onion and stir some more.

Set the avocados on a serving plate, cut side up. Spoon the salmon mixture on to each avocado, covering generously. Sprinkle with the dried parsley, scatter some watercress around to decorate, and serve.

Variation: for an extra-smoky taste, sprinkle each serving with half a teaspoon of smoked paprika.

PEPPERED MACKEREL AND ROCKET PÂTÉ ON TOASTED RYE BREAD

A quick alternative to cooked fish, tasty for breakfast, lunch or supper.

Serves 2
Preparation time: 7 minutes
Cooking time: None
Total: 7 minutes
Suggested days: any
Net carbs per serving: 2g
Protein per serving: 5g

200g peppered mackerel
1 tsp lime juice
2 tbsp extra-virgin olive oil
½ tsp tamari soy sauce
1 tbsp soy lecithin granules
1 shitake mushroom
1 spring onion
50g rocket
4 slices pumpernickel-type rye bread
1 tsp dried parsley

Skin and flake the mackerel into a food processor. Add the lime juice, olive oil, tamari, soy lecithin, mushroom and spring onion and blend until smooth.

Either add the rocket to the rest of the ingredients and blend it in for a lusciously green spreading pâté, or if you prefer a crunchy texture, chop the rocket and the green stems of the spring onion very finely and stir into the paste.

Toast the rye bread and spread the pâté on it luxuriantly. Finally, sprinkle with the parsley.

CAJUN SWEET POTATO WEDGES

You'll ditch the chips once you've tried these. Serve with a main dish, or eat on their own!

Serves 4
Preparation time: 5 minutes
Cooking time: 40 minutes
Total: 45 minutes
Suggested days: high- or low-carb

Net carbs per serving: 25g
Protein per serving: 1g

**4 medium-sized sweet potatoes, peeled and sliced
  into wedges
extra-virgin olive oil spray
Cajun spice mix**

Preheat the oven to 200°C.

Blanch the potato wedges in a pan of boiling water until they are soft enough to put a fork into, but not so soft they fall apart.

Spray a shallow baking tray with a little olive oil, and heat it in the oven.

Once the wedges are ready, drain in a colander and put them on the tray, turning them in the oil to cover. Lightly dust the wedges with the Cajun spices, then bake them in the oven for 20 minutes on each side, or until brown and crispy.

GARLIC AND CORIANDER SAUCE

The perfect accompaniment to any fish dish.

Serves 2
Preparation time: 5 minutes
Cooking time: None
Total: 5 minutes
Suggested days: any
Net carbs per serving: 0g
Protein per serving: 0g

4 cloves of garlic, peeled and finely chopped
a large handful of coriander, stalks removed
1 tbsp extra-virgin olive oil

Chop the garlic and coriander very finely, then put them into a bowl with the olive oil and mix together until well blended. Chill in the refrigerator for 1 hour before serving.

Drizzle over cod, tuna or any other fish and enjoy the flavours!

This mixture keeps well for a few days in the refrigerator.

TOMATO SOUP WITH FENNEL AND SWEET POTATO

A warming, hearty soup – ideal as a starter.

Serves 2
Preparation time: 10 minutes
Cooking time: 1 hour
Total: 1 hour 10 minutes
Suggested days: high- or low-carb
Net carbs per serving: 26.5g
Protein per serving: 4.5g

extra-virgin olive oil spray
1 large onion, peeled and sliced
2 large fennel bulbs, finely sliced
1 small sweet potato, peeled and diced
400ml tinned tomatoes, chopped
1 bay leaf
4 tomatoes, skinned, deseeded and chopped
½ tsp fresh dill, snipped
a few dill sprigs to garnish

Heat a few squirts of olive oil in a large saucepan over a medium heat. Add the onion and fennel and cook for 3–4 minutes, stirring occasionally until the vegetables begin to soften.

Add the sweet potato, tinned tomatoes, bay leaf and about 850ml water, and season with salt to taste.

Bring to the boil, reduce the heat, cover and simmer for 25–30 minutes, stirring occasionally.

Allow the soup to cool slightly, then transfer to a blender and process until smooth. (If the soup contains a lot of liquid, drain some of this off for blending, then re-add to the blended mixture.)

Return the soup to the saucepan, stir in the chopped tomatoes and dill and simmer gently for 10 minutes.

Serve in warmed bowls, garnish with dill and freshly ground black pepper and enjoy!

POTAJE DE GARBANZOS CON CALAMARES (CALAMARI AND CHICKPEA SOUP)

A protein-packed Mediterranean speciality. Ask your fishmonger to prepare the squid for you, or you can buy ready-prepared packs from the fishmonger's counter at larger supermarkets.

Serves 2
Preparation time: 10 minutes
Cooking time: 30 minutes
Total: 40 minutes
Suggested days: high- or low-carb
Net carbs per serving: 26.5g
Protein per serving: 45g

50ml extra-virgin olive oil
1 red and 1 green pepper, diced
1 medium onion, peeled and finely chopped
¼ tsp saffron strands
1 tsp sweet paprika
500g fresh squid, prepared and sliced
300g chickpeas, drained and rinsed

In a medium-size pan, heat the olive oil and add the peppers and onion. Fry gently for about 10 minutes, then add the saffron and paprika, stir, and fry for a further minute. Add the squid, the chickpeas, and 2 litres of water.

Put the pan on a high heat, bring to the boil, reduce the heat and simmer for 10 minutes.

TZATZIKI

A popular Greek dip that works perfectly with grilled meat and vegetables. It also goes well with brown pitta on high-carb days.

Serves 4
Preparation time: 20 minutes
Cooking time: None
Total: 20 minutes
Suggested days: high- or low-carb
Net carbs per serving: 7g
Protein per serving: 8g

3 tbsp extra-virgin olive oil
juice of ¼ lemon
1 tbsp balsamic vinegar

½ tsp salt
½ tsp freshly ground black pepper
2 cloves of garlic, peeled and finely chopped
240ml natural, live Greek yoghurt
2 cucumbers, peeled, deseeded and finely diced
1 tsp chopped fresh dill

Mix the olive oil, lemon juice, vinegar, salt, pepper and garlic together in a bowl until combined. Add the yoghurt and mix well. Add the cucumber and chopped dill, then chill for 2–3 hours in the refrigerator before serving.

FRUIT AND FIBRE YOGHURT POT

This is a really tasty, healthy breakfast. It's also a great alternative to ice cream.

Serves 1
Preparation time: 2 minutes
Cooking time: None
Total: 2 minutes
Suggested days: high- or low-carb
Net carbs per serving: 16g
Protein per serving: 9g

2 tbsp natural, live Greek yoghurt
2 tbsp rolled oats
a handful of fresh blueberries

Simply spoon the yoghurt into a bowl and sprinkle with the oats and berries.

Fish

COD STEAKS WITH GARLIC AND SAFFRON AIOLI

A wonderfully healthy and hearty meal, ideal for the slow cooker.

Serves 4
Preparation time: 30 minutes
Cooking time: 90 minutes (slow cooker), 30 minutes (oven)
Total: 2 hours (slow cooker), 1 hour (oven)
Suggested days: any
Net carbs per serving: 2g
Protein per serving: 36.5g

for the aioli:
2 large cloves of garlic, peeled
¼ tsp saffron strands
1 egg yolk
200ml extra-virgin olive oil
2 tbsp lemon juice

for the marinade:
2 tbsp extra-virgin olive oil
4 cloves of garlic, peeled and finely chopped
1 red onion, peeled and finely chopped
1 tbsp chopped parsley
2 tbsp chopped thyme

4 sprigs fresh rosemary
1 lemon, sliced
4 × 150g thick cod fillets, skin on

To make the aioli, crush the garlic and saffron in a pestle and mortar to form a paste. Put in a blender, add the egg yolk and blend for 30 seconds. Then with the blender on slow, gradually add the olive oil until the paste becomes smooth and thick. Spoon into a bowl and stir in the lemon juice.

Cover and put in the fridge.

To make the marinade, mix the olive oil, garlic, onion, parsley and thyme in a bowl and leave to infuse for 10–15 minutes.

If you're cooking this in a conventional oven, preheat it now to 180°C.

Put the rosemary and lemon slices in the base of a casserole or in the slow cooker and drizzle over a little more olive oil. Add the cod, skin-side up. Pour the marinade over the fish and cover with the lid.

If you're using a slow cooker, switch to 'high' and cook for 30 minutes, then switch to 'auto' and cook for a further hour, or until the cod is cooked through.

If you're cooking conventionally, bake the cod in the oven for 30 minutes or until it is cooked through.

Serve with the saffron aioli and steamed green vegetables.

STUFFED MEDITERRANEAN PEPPERS WITH PRAWNS

A simple dish that's full of flavour and looks impressive.

Serves 4
Preparation time: 20 minutes
Cooking time: 30 minutes
Total: 50 minutes
Suggested days: high- or low-carb

Net carbs per serving: 13.5g
Protein per serving: 29.5g

4 red peppers
50ml extra-virgin olive oil
400g peeled king prawns (raw or ready cooked)
8 medium tomatoes, diced
1 medium onion, peeled and finely chopped
1 large chilli, finely chopped

Preheat the oven to 210°C.

Chop the lids off the peppers and reserve for later. Trim the base of the peppers to form a flat surface, being careful not to make holes through them. Using a spoon, remove the seeds and white fleshy inners. Place the peppers upright in a roasting dish and drizzle with some of the olive oil. Bake in the preheated oven for 15 minutes.

In the meantime, heat a frying pan with a little olive oil, and if using raw prawns, fry them gently until they turn pink. Otherwise just put the prawns into the pan, then add the tomatoes, onion and chilli and continue to cook for 12–15 minutes on a low-medium heat, stirring periodically. Season to taste.

Remove the peppers from the oven (if you have not already done so) and fill them with the contents of the frying pan.

Put the lids back on the peppers and return to the oven. Bake for a further 10–15 minutes until soft and lightly browned.

Serve with a side salad.

MONKFISH CURRY

....

A deliciously chunky curry that's full of goodness.

Serves 4
Preparation time: 15 minutes
Cooking time: 4 hours 30 minutes
Total time: 4 hours 45 minutes
Suggested days: high-carb
Net carbs per serving: 37g
Protein per serving: 44g

4 tbsp extra-virgin olive oil
1 large onion, peeled and finely chopped
1 tbsp curry powder, or to taste
6 tinned tomatoes, chopped
extra-virgin olive oil spray
500g monkfish tail fillets, trimmed and cut into
   bite-sized chunks
400g green or black lentils, drained and rinsed
400g chickpeas, drained and rinsed
4 medium carrots, peeled and diced
200g baked beans
500ml fish stock
200g cooked prawns

Heat the extra-virgin olive oil in a large saucepan over a medium heat.

Add the onion and fry until golden-brown. Add the curry powder and fry for 1 minute. Finally, add the tomatoes and cook for a further 5–10 minutes.

Spray a shallow pan with olive oil and lightly fry the monk-fish over a low heat for 5 minutes.

Add the monkfish and cooking juices to the tomato-onion mix in the saucepan and cook for a further minute or until lightly golden.

Add the lentils, chickpeas, carrots and baked beans. Stir well and cook for 1 minute.

Add the fish stock, bring to a simmer, and leave with a lid on over a very low heat for 4 hours, stirring occasionally.

Ten minutes before serving, add the prawns.

Serve with vegetables and/or brown rice.

THAI FISH CAKES

Who said fish cakes can't be Pyramid-approved?!

Serves 4
Preparation time: 5 minutes
Cooking time: 15 minutes
Total: 20 minutes
Suggested days: high- or low-carb
Net carbs per serving: 14g
Protein per serving: 25g

4 shallots, peeled and quartered
3cm fresh ginger, peeled and roughly chopped
3 cloves of garlic, peeled and crushed
a handful of fresh coriander (stalks on)
1 medium chilli, deseeded and finely chopped
550g cod or monkfish fillet, cut into chunks
2 tbsp tamari soy sauce
1 egg white

2 tbsp plain wholemeal flour
zest and juice of 1 lime
extra-virgin olive oil spray

Put the shallots, ginger, garlic, coriander and chilli in a blender and pulse until roughly chopped.

Add the fish and pulse again until well mixed. Stop before it becomes a smooth paste. Transfer to a large mixing bowl and add the soy sauce, egg white, flour, lime zest and juice. Combine by hand to mix all the ingredients.

Divide the fish mixture into individual cakes, then heat a few squirts of olive oil in a non-stick frying pan and fry the cakes for 3–4 minutes on each side until golden-brown and cooked through.

Serve with salad.

ANDALUCIAN-STYLE SEA BASS

A Spanish dish that'll blow you away. The fabulous sauce can be used in a variety of dishes.

Serves 2
Preparation time: 10 minutes
Cooking time: 30 minutes
Total: 40 minutes
Suggested days: high- or low-carb
Net carbs per serving: 12g
Protein per serving: 22.5g

extra-virgin olive oil spray
2 cloves of garlic, peeled and crushed
1 small onion, peeled and finely chopped

1 red and 1 green pepper, deseeded and finely
   chopped
200g fresh or tinned tomatoes, finely chopped
1 tsp chopped thyme
2 × 150g sea bass fillets (or cod or dorada if
   preferred)

Preheat your oven to 200°C.

In a non-stick frying pan, heat a few squirts of olive oil and fry the garlic, onion and pepper for 6–7 minutes, stirring regularly.

Add the chopped tomatoes to the pan and fry for a further 2 minutes.

Sprinkle in the thyme, then remove from the heat and set to one side.

Spray a baking dish with olive oil and bake the sea bass in the preheated oven for about 10 minutes.

Remove the fish once it is cooked through (thick fillets may need an extra minute or two). Coat the fillets with the sauce, return to the oven and bake for a further 10 minutes.

SEARED TUNA WITH SESAME SEEDS

A deliciously light Pyramid favourite.

Serves 4
Preparation time: 30 minutes
Cooking time: 10 minutes
Total: 40 minutes
Suggested days: any
Net carbs per serving: 5g
Protein per serving: 53g

for the marinade:
4 tbsp tamari soy sauce
1 tbsp wasabi paste
2cm fresh ginger, peeled and grated
2 tbsp brown-rice vinegar

800g tuna, sliced into thick strips
400g pak choi
1 tbsp sesame oil
400g bean sprouts
2 cloves of garlic, peeled and finely chopped
125g sesame seeds
extra-virgin olive oil spray

In a deep dish large enough to take the tuna, mix the soy sauce, wasabi, ginger and vinegar. Marinade the tuna slices in the mixture for 15 minutes on each side, ensuring they are well coated.

In the meantime, trim the bases from the pak choi and slice in half lengthways. Steam for approximately 3 minutes.

Heat the sesame oil in a non-stick wok over a medium heat. Add the bean sprouts and fry for 1–2 minutes. Add the pak choi and garlic, and fry for a further minute. Set aside and keep warm.

Remove the tuna from the marinade and coat with the sesame seeds on both sides. In a clean pan on a high heat put a few squirts of olive oil and sear the tuna for 1–2 minutes on each side.

Place the bean sprouts and pak choi on plates and top with the seared tuna. Add a little more tamari soy sauce to serve if you wish.

Meat, Poultry and Game

BENJIE'S SLOW COOKER BEEF STEW

You won't believe this delicious stew is Pyramid-approved. It's also great reheated.

Serves 4
Preparation time: 15 minutes
Cooking time: 6–8 hours/overnight
Total: 8 hours 15 minutes
Suggested day: high-carb
Net carbs per serving: 39g
Protein per serving: 31g

500g lean stewing steak
extra-virgin olive oil spray
2 onions, peeled and chopped
2 leeks, trimmed, rinsed and sliced
1 turnip, peeled and diced
4 medium sweet potatoes, peeled and diced
6 carrots, peeled and diced
200g kidney beans, drained and rinsed
freshly ground black pepper
500ml stock or water

Turn your slow cooker to 'high'. When it's heated, brown the steak and vegetables in the olive oil. Add the kidney beans, season with pepper to taste, pour over 500ml stock or water, and set cooker to 'low'.

Cook for 6–8 hours, or overnight.

If you want to make it the conventional way, heat the oil in a large heavy-based pan, brown the steak then remove and set aside. Add a few more sprays of oil to the same pan and gently soften the vegetables in the order listed, then return the meat to the pan. Increase the heat and add the stock or water and beans. Bring to the boil, lower the heat and simmer as gently as possible for 2 hours.

CHILLI CON CARNE

A family favourite – Pyramid style!

Serves 4
Preparation time: 15 minutes
Cooking time: 45 minutes
Total: 1 hour
Suggested days: high-carb
Net carbs per serving: 64g (with pitta bread)
Protein per serving: 37g

extra-virgin olive oil spray
1 large onion, finely chopped
1 clove of garlic, peeled and finely chopped
500g lean minced beef
2 tsp medium chilli powder
1 tsp ground cumin
400g tomatoes, chopped
300ml beef stock
1 red pepper, deseeded and finely diced
400g kidney beans, drained and rinsed
brown pitta bread or brown rice to serve

Put about 5 sprays of olive oil in a large saucepan on a medium heat, and soften the onion and garlic, stirring periodically, for about 5 minutes.

Turn up the heat, add the beef and brown it all over. Reduce the heat, add the chilli powder and cumin and cook for a further minute. Add the chopped tomatoes and the stock, then simmer gently over a low heat for 30 minutes.

Add the red pepper and kidney beans and simmer for a further 10 minutes.

Season to taste and serve with brown rice or brown pitta bread.

SPAGHETTI BOLOGNESE

Another family favourite that won't pack on the pounds.

Serves 4
Preparation time: 15 minutes
Cooking time: 30 minutes
Total: 45 minutes
Suggested days: high- or low-carb
Net carbs per serving: 22g
Protein per serving: 36g

extra-virgin olive oil spray
500g lean minced beef
2 large onions, peeled and finely chopped
200g courgette, finely chopped
1 red pepper, deseeded and finely chopped
125g button mushrooms, sliced
2 cloves of garlic, peeled and finely chopped

400g cherry tomatoes, fresh or tinned
200ml beef stock
400g wholewheat spaghetti
grated low-fat cheese to serve

Put about 5 sprays of oil into a pan over a medium heat. Once the oil is hot, add the mince and fry until browned. Then add the onion, courgette, pepper and button mushrooms and cook over medium heat for a further 3–4 minutes.

Add the garlic, turn down the heat and cook for 4–5 minutes, stirring periodically until the juices start to thicken.

Add the cherry tomatoes and beef stock, stir, then put a lid on the pan and simmer gently for 20 minutes, stirring occasionally.

Cook the spaghetti according to packet instructions. To prevent the spaghetti sticking together, you can add a few squirts of olive oil to the water.

Drain the spaghetti and serve with the sauce on top. Sprinkle with a little grated low-fat cheese if desired.

SPICY MEATBALLS

A cosy classic with a hint of heat.

Makes 12–16 meatballs
Preparation time: 5 minutes
Cooking time: 20 minutes
Total time: 25 minutes
Suggested days: high- or low-carb
Net carbs per serving (4 meatballs): 10g
Protein per serving (4 meatballs): 32g

50g oats
1 tbsp low-fat Parmesan, grated
¼ onion, peeled and finely chopped
1 clove of garlic, peeled and finely chopped
1 medium-heat red chilli, deseeded and very finely
   chopped
¼ tsp dried or ½ tbsp chopped fresh oregano
¼ tsp dried or ½ tbsp chopped fresh thyme
freshly ground black pepper to taste
1 egg (optional)
450g lean minced beef
extra-virgin olive oil spray

If you prefer to cook these in the oven, preheat it now to 180°C.

Put all the ingredients except the mince and olive oil into a large bowl. Mix well, then add the mince and mix again.

Form the mixture into meatballs and then either heat some olive oil in a non-stick pan and fry them until browned and cooked through, or bake in the preheated oven on a lightly oiled baking tray for 15–20 minutes, turning occasionally.

SUNDRIED BEEFBURGERS

A delicious twist on a favourite dish.

Makes 4 burgers
Preparation time: 10 minutes
Cooking time: 15 minutes
Total: 25 minutes
Suggested days: high- or low-carb

Net carbs per burger: 31g
Protein per burger: 3g

500g lean minced beef
1 medium onion, peeled and finely chopped
6 sundried tomatoes, finely chopped
1 egg
1 tsp Cajun spice mix

to serve:
granary or wholemeal burger buns
a few slices of tomato

Mix all the burger ingredients together in a bowl. Divide the mixture into four and mould into burger shapes, firming each one well to prevent them falling apart during cooking. Refrigerate for an hour to help bind.

Grill under a medium heat for 6–8 minutes on each side. Alternatively, cook on the barbeque.

COURGETTES STUFFED WITH MINCED LAMB

A wonderfully light lunch or dinner with bundles of flavour.

Serves 2
Preparation time: 10 minutes
Cooking time: 20 minutes
Total: 30 minutes
Suggested days: any
Net carbs per serving: 5g
Protein per serving: 26g

for the stuffing:
extra-virgin olive oil spray
200g lean lamb mince
a handful of fresh mint, finely chopped
a handful of fresh thyme, finely chopped
a sprinkling of finely chopped fresh or dried
    oregano
1 large onion, peeled and finely chopped
2 cloves of garlic, peeled and finely chopped

2 courgettes, halved lengthways and hollowed out

Preheat oven to 170°C.

Spray a little olive oil into a frying pan on a medium heat, and brown the lamb.

Add the remaining stuffing ingredients and fry for a further 2 minutes, until the flavours have infused.

Put the courgette halves on to a baking tray, and spoon the stuffing mixture into them. Press down firmly with the back of a spoon to ensure the courgettes are well packed.

Bake in the preheated oven for 20 minutes.

SMOKED LENTIL, SEAWEED AND TURKEY CASSEROLE

This hearty casserole is a great dish full of fibre and mood-balancing nutrients to beat the change-of-season blues. It's also rich in iodine so it will help speed up your metabolism.

Serves 4
Preparation time: 35 minutes
Cooking time: 25 minutes

Total: 1 hour
Suggested days: any
Net carbs per serving: 6g
Protein per serving: 7g

extra-virgin olive oil spray
4 medium red onions, peeled and finely chopped
4 spring onions, finely chopped
5 cloves of garlic, peeled and finely chopped
3 medium carrots, peeled and finely chopped
1 small sweet potato, peeled and finely chopped
300g turkey breast fillets, chopped into bitesize
  pieces
1 tbsp garam masala powder
20g arame seaweed
400g tinned lentils
2 tbsp soy lecithin granules
100g baby-leaf spinach
1 tsp hot smoked paprika

Heat about 5 sprays of olive oil in a large pan, then put in the onion, spring onion, garlic, carrot and sweet potato and cook over a low heat, stirring often, for about 5 minutes.

Add the turkey breast, season to taste and cook for 2–3 minutes until golden-brown. Add the garam masala and half a cup of water and let the vegetables steam in the juices for 5 minutes.

Crush the seaweed a little so that it breaks into small pieces and add to the pan, together with the lentils. Let it steam over a low heat for another 5 minutes.

Add the soy lecithin and a bit more water if it needs it, stir and allow to simmer for 15 minutes.

Then just add the baby spinach and paprika, stir and leave the casserole to rest for another 15–20 minutes to let the flavours infuse just a little longer.

TURKEY MEATBALLS ITALIAN STYLE

A classic with a turkey twist.

Makes 12–16 meatballs
Preparation time: 5 minutes
Cooking time: 20 minutes
Total: 25 minutes
Suggested days: high- or low-carb
Net carbs per serving: 12g
Protein per serving: 44g

50g rolled oats
1 tbsp grated low-fat Parmesan cheese
¼ onion, peeled and finely chopped
¼ green pepper, deseeded and finely chopped
1 clove of garlic, peeled and finely chopped
¼ tsp dried or ½ tbsp chopped fresh oregano
¼ tsp dried or ½ tbsp chopped fresh thyme
freshly ground black pepper
1 egg (optional)
450g lean turkey mince
extra-virgin olive oil spray

If you prefer to cook these in the oven, preheat it now to 200°C.

Mix all the ingredients except the turkey and olive oil together in a large bowl. Add the turkey, blend well and form the mixture into 12–16 meatballs.

Now either heat a couple of sprays of olive oil in a non-stick pan, then fry the balls until browned on the outside and cooked through, or cook in the oven on a lightly oiled baking tray for 15–20 minutes, turning occasionally.

SPANISH CHICKEN

A simple dish that'll sweep your taste buds off your tongue!

Serves 2
Preparation time: 10 minutes
Cooking time: 40 minutes
Total: 50 minutes
Suggested days: any
Net carbs per serving: 6g
Protein per serving: 34g

2 × 150g chicken breasts
6 green olives, finely sliced
4 small vine tomatoes, finely sliced
6 button mushrooms, finely sliced
1 small red onion, peeled and finely chopped
4 cloves of garlic, peeled and finely chopped
a pinch of dried chilli
4 slices Parma ham (fat removed)
green beans to serve

Preheat the oven to 200°C.

Create a pocket in each chicken breast by slicing them lengthways, being careful not to cut right through.

In a bowl, mix the olives, tomatoes, mushrooms, onion, garlic and chilli. Stuff the chicken breasts with this mixture, then wrap 2 slices of Parma ham tightly around each breast and wrap them each in foil to secure.

Place on a baking tray and cook for 25–30 minutes in the oven until the chicken is cooked through. When it is, remove the foil and cook for a further 5–10 minutes until lightly browned.

Green beans are particularly good with this dish, but any similar green vegetable will work well.

Variation: if you like a bit more kick, use olives stuffed with red chilli.

VENISON STIR-FRY WITH VEGETABLES

A quick and simple light lunch or evening meal that (with quantities increased) would also make a great dinner party dish.

Serves 2
Preparation time: 15 minutes
Cooking time: 10 minutes
Total: 25 minutes
Suggested days: any
Net carbs per serving: 4g
Protein per serving: 36g

extra-virgin olive oil spray
300g venison, cut into small strips
200g pak choi, trimmed and chopped
1 leek, trimmed, washed and cut into fine strips
½ yellow and ½ red pepper, deseeded and finely sliced

2 spring onions, finely chopped
10 button mushrooms, sliced
1 medium-heat red chilli, finely chopped
1 tbsp tamari soy sauce

Heat about 10 sprays of oil in a wok over a medium-high heat.

Once the oil is hot, add the venison and stir-fry for 1–2 minutes until lightly browned.

Add the pak choi, leek, peppers, spring onion and mushrooms. Stir-fry for a further 6 minutes, stirring frequently.

Add the chilli and soy sauce and continue to fry for a further 2–3 minutes.

PAN-FRIED PHEASANT WITH SALSA VERDE AND SWEET POTATO MASH

A deliciously different and easy high-protein dish.

Serves 2
Preparation time: 30 minutes
Cooking time: 15 minutes
Total: 45 minutes
Suggested days: high- or low-carb
Net carbs per serving: 29g
Protein per serving: 60g

for the sweet potato mash:
2 sweet potatoes, peeled and quartered
½ tbsp skimmed milk
freshly ground black pepper

for the salsa verde:
4 cloves of garlic, peeled and finely chopped
1 tbsp capers, drained
8 anchovy fillets, drained and chopped
a handful of flat-leafed parsley
a handful of basil leaves
2 tsp Dijon mustard
2 tbsp rice vinegar
4 tbsp extra-virgin olive oil
freshly ground black pepper

4 skinless pheasant breasts
2 tbsp extra-virgin olive oil
freshly ground black pepper

First bring the sweet potatoes to the boil in a covered sauce-pan, then simmer for 15–20 minutes or until soft.

To make the salsa verde, put the garlic, capers, anchovy fillets, herbs, mustard and 1 tablespoon of the rice vinegar into a food processor. Whizz together until the ingredients have blended and are roughly chopped. Stir in the remaining rice vinegar and extra-virgin olive oil. Season with black pepper, then cover and leave to mature.

For the pheasant, heat the olive oil in a non-stick frying pan over a medium-high heat. Season the pheasant breasts on both sides, then lightly fry for 2–3 minutes on each side.

Once the sweet potatoes are soft, drain them and add the skimmed milk. Mash until smooth and creamy, then add black pepper to season.

Serve the pheasant on the sweet potato mash and top with the salsa verde.

PHEASANT AND HAZELNUT SALAD

Because salad doesn't have to be boring!

Serves 6
Preparation time: 15 minutes
Cooking time: 45 minutes
Total: 1 hour
Suggested days: any
Net carbs per serving: 2g
Protein per serving: 30g

1 whole pheasant
extra-virgin olive oil spray
4 tbsp hazelnuts
400g mixed salad leaves (e.g., spinach, chicory,
  rocket and watercress)
2 tbsp extra-virgin olive oil
2 tbsp brown rice vinegar

Preheat the oven to 200°C.

Lightly spray the pheasant with olive oil, season with salt and freshly ground pepper and roast in the oven for 45 minutes.

Pull a leg away from the bird to test if it's ready. It should be slightly bloody, but not blue. When cooked to your liking, remove the bird from the oven, cover in foil and leave to rest for 15 minutes.

While it's resting, lightly toast the hazelnuts in a spray or two of olive oil, either in the oven or in a frying pan.

Carve the pheasant and cut the meat into strips. Set it to one side and cover to keep warm.

Wash and dry your salad leaves, then roughly chop them.

Crush the hazelnuts roughly in a pestle and mortar, or wrap in a cloth and crush with a rolling pin.

In a large salad bowl, toss the pheasant strips and nuts together using your hands. Add the olive oil, vinegar and a little juice from the roasting tray.

Divide the salad leaves evenly between 6 plates and top with the pheasant and nut mixture.

Vegetarian Dishes

GOOD-CARB STEAM FRY

This delicious 'steam fry' is quick and easy, packed with nutrients and makes a filling low-fat, low-carb meal.

Serves 3
Preparation time: 5 minutes
Cooking time: 15 minutes
Total: 20 minutes
Suggested days: any
Net carbs per serving: 5g
Total protein per serving: 5g

extra-virgin olive oil spray
100g shitake mushrooms, wiped and sliced
100g pak choi, chard or baby-leaf spinach, roughly chopped
150g tenderstem broccoli
4 spring onions, sliced
2 cloves of garlic, peeled and finely chopped

4 tbsp olive oil

2 tbsp soy lecithin granules

½ tsp korma curry mix or 1 tbsp soy sauce

100g tinned lentils, drained and rinsed, or
  frozen peas

200g soy-bean sprouts

Heat a couple of sprays of oil in a deep non-stick pan or wok on a medium heat, then add the mushrooms, pak choi, broccoli, spring onions and garlic.

Stir gently, and add the 4 tablespoons of olive oil, salt to taste, the soy lecithin and the curry powder or soy sauce, depending on your preference.

Keep stirring gently for a couple of minutes, then add about a quarter of a cup of hot water. Put the lid on the pan and leave the vegetables to steam in their own juice for 5 minutes.

In the meantime, if you're using frozen peas defrost them gently in another pan so when you add them they don't bring the temperature down too low.

After 5 minutes, add the lentils or peas and the soy-bean sprouts and stir a little more. If the vegetables look too dry, add a little more water. Cover and let it simmer on a very low heat for another 5 minutes. Stir one last time.

If you're really hungry and can't wait, you can eat now, but if you're not in such a rush, cover again and let the steam continue to work its magic for another 5–10 minutes, so it continues to bring out the flavours of the ingredients.

CHICKPEA BALTI

···

An energising vegetarian meal that's easy to make.

Serves 2
Preparation time: 20 minutes
Cooking time: 20 minutes
Total: 40 minutes
Suggested days: high-carb
Net carbs per serving: 40.5g
Protein per serving: 11g

for the sauce:
extra-virgin olive oil spray
1 large onion, peeled and finely chopped
1 clove of garlic, peeled and finely chopped
**2½cm fresh ginger, peeled and finely chopped
    or grated**
4 tsp medium curry paste, or to taste
400g chopped tomatoes
a large handful of coriander, finely chopped

a handful of cauliflower florets
1 large onion, peeled and cut into chunks
1 sweet potato, peeled and diced
1 courgette, sliced
1 red pepper, deseeded and roughly chopped
200g chickpeas, drained and rinsed
a handful of peas (fresh or frozen)
a handful of fresh coriander, chopped

Heat a couple of sprays of olive oil in a large heavy pan over a medium heat. Add the the onion, garlic and ginger and sweat for a few minutes, stirring often.

Add the curry paste, tomatoes and coriander and simmer for a further 10 minutes.

Meanwhile, in another pan steam the cauliflower, onion, sweet potato, courgette and pepper until soft. Tip the steamed vegetables into the pan containing the sauce and mix in the chickpeas, peas and coriander.

Cook gently for a further 5 minutes.

CHICKPEA SUMMER SALAD

A light summer recipe that's packed with good stuff. This is best served 12–24 hours after preparation.

Serves 4
Preparation time: 10 minutes
Cooking time: 5 minutes
Total: 15 minutes
Suggested days: high- or low-carb
Net carbs per serving: 17g
Protein per serving: 7.5g

for the dressing:
2 tbsp extra-virgin olive oil
1 tbsp freshly squeezed lemon juice
2 tbsp balsamic vinegar
1 clove of garlic, peeled and finely chopped

200g chickpeas, drained and rinsed

75g broccoli florets, parboiled, drained and cooled
1 medium red onion, peeled and diced
3 tbsp finely chopped fresh parsley
1 tbsp finely chopped fresh basil

Put the olive oil, lemon, balsamic vinegar and garlic in a bowl and season with salt and black pepper to taste. Mix well to allow the flavours to infuse.

In a salad bowl, toss the chickpeas, broccoli, onion and herbs together. Pour over the dressing and toss again.

Cover and place in the refrigerator for 12–24 hours, stirring every so often to help the salad marinate evenly.

Serve on top of large lettuce leaves.

BLACK BEAN CHILLI

A vegetarian twist on a classic dish.

Serves 4
Preparation time: 8 hours + 30 minutes
Cooking time: 90 minutes
Total: 8 + 2 hours
Suggested days: high- or low-carb
Net carbs per serving: 17g
Protein per serving: 7g

700g black beans
4 tbsp brown-rice vinegar
2 onions, peeled and finely chopped
4 cloves of garlic, peeled and finely chopped
1 bay leaf
1 green pepper, roughly chopped

2 tsp ground cumin
½ tsp cayenne pepper
1 tbsp sweet paprika
2 tbsp chilli powder
2 tsp oregano
400g tinned tomatoes

Cover the beans with cold water and leave to soak for 8 hours or overnight.

When you're ready to cook, drain the beans and set aside.

Heat a large pan over medium-high heat, add 2 table-spoons of the vinegar and sauté half the onion and half the garlic for about 5 minutes, stirring all the time. Add the black beans, 2 litres of water and the bay leaf. Bring to the boil, then cover and simmer for an hour.

Meanwhile, in a second large pan heat the rest of the vinegar and sauté the remaining onion and garlic until soft. Add the green pepper and continue to sauté until slightly soft. Add the spices and herbs and sauté for a further 3–5 minutes. You may need to add a little water to stop things sticking. Finally, add the tomatoes and their juice and simmer for another 30 minutes.

Once the black beans have simmered for an hour, drain and add them to the tomato mixture. Simmer everything together for 30 minutes. Discard the bay leaf.

If desired, you can simmer for an extra 1–2 hours or until the chilli reaches the desired consistency.

Serve with wholemeal pitta, salad or brown rice.

Desserts

ALMOND BUTTER COOKIES

Nutty and buttery, with a very low GL.

Makes 6–8 cookies
Preparation time: 5 minutes
Cooking time: 12 minutes
Total: 17 minutes
Suggested days: high- or low-carb
Net carbs per cookie: 4g
Protein per cookie: 5g

225g almond butter
1 egg
190g xylitol
50g walnut pieces
50g hazelnuts

Preheat the oven to 180°C.

Put all the ingredients into a food processor and blitz until thoroughly mixed.

Line a baking tray with greaseproof paper and place spoonfuls of the mixture on to it, leaving enough space for them to spread a little.

Bake in the oven for 10–12 minutes or until the tops look crispy-brown.

Cool and enjoy!

MOST AWESOME DELICIOUS HEALTHY CHEESECAKE

Can you believe it's not bad for you?! You'll find protein powder in health stores, online or in large supermarkets, and jelly crystals in any large supermarket.

Serves 4
Preparation time: 20 minutes
Cooking time: 30 minutes
Total: 50 minutes
Suggested days: high- or low-carb
Net carbs per serving: 21g
Protein per serving: 26g with protein powder or 17g without

for the base:
75g peanut butter
75g oatmeal
non-stick cooking spray (optional)

for the topping:
125g fat-free cream cheese
200g fat-free natural Greek yoghurt
1 large scoop of strawberry protein powder (optional)
1 × sachet sugar-free strawberry jelly crystals
a few strawberries to decorate

a round, loose-based tin approx. 23cm diameter × 4cm deep

Preheat your oven to 150°C.

Put the peanut butter into a bowl and warm it for about 15 seconds in the microwave, then stir in the oatmeal until it's well mixed and sticks together nicely.

Line the cheesecake tin with greaseproof paper or one squirt of non-stick cooking spray to stop the base sticking. Tip in your mixture and use a fork to pat it down and spread it out. Cook the base in the preheated oven for 10 minutes, or until the top starts to go a deeper brown. Leave to cool.

Next the topping: this takes about 2 minutes, so make sure you've allowed your base 15 minutes to cool before you start.

In a mixing bowl put the cream cheese and yoghurt, plus protein powder if you want to use it. No need to mix them yet.

Make up the jelly to about 500ml (half you'd normally make). Whilst it's still warm, tip it into the mixing bowl with the other ingredients. Whisk it all together until smooth. Immediately pour over the cheesecake base – this mixture sets very quickly!

Slice the strawberries and decorate the top of your cheese-cake, then put it in the fridge to set. It should be ready in 15 minutes.

Remove it from the tin, cut yourself a quarter and enjoy!

CHOCOLATE PROTEIN-PACKED BROWNIES

A heavenly treat that's safe to eat!

Makes 8–10 brownies
Preparation time: 10 minutes
Cooking time: 30 minutes
Total: 40 minutes
Suggested days: high- or low-carb

Net carbs per serving: 8g
Protein per serving: 4g

125g brown soy flour
2 scoops vanilla protein powder
½ tsp baking powder
60g xylitol
25g cocoa powder
5 egg whites
120ml water
60g blueberries, blended
sunflower oil, Cake Release or similar for oiling
    the tin
a baking tin approx. 20cm × 20cm

Preheat the oven to 190°C.

Put the dry ingredients into a large bowl. Mix the wet ingredients together in a medium-sized bowl, then add them to the dry and mix well.

Lightly oil the tin and pour in the batter. Bake for 20–30 minutes in the oven.

Cut into squares and leave to cool.

ORGANIC CHOCOLATE COOKIES

These cookies are fabulous, with a silly-low GL. Of course the ingredients don't *all* have to be organic, but use as much organic as you can. You may wonder why this recipe allows butter when it is not on the list of Pyramid-approved foods. This is a very rare exception for a recipe that has been devised personally by Miguel, but please don't think it is OK to use elsewhere! Cacao nibs can be bought at health-food stores.

Makes 8–10 cookies
Preparation time: 10 minutes
Cooking time: 8 minutes
Total: 18 minutes
Suggested days: high- or low-carb
Net carbs per cookie: 8g
Protein per cookie: 3g

250g plain organic wholewheat flour
½ tsp salt
1 tsp baking powder
150g xylitol
110g organic cocoa powder
100g raw cacao nibs
120g organic pecans or other nuts
280g organic butter
2 organic eggs
1 tsp organic vanilla extract (optional)

Preheat your oven to 180°C.

Combine the flour, salt and baking powder in a bowl and mix well. Add the rest of the dry ingredients and mix.

In another bowl cream the butter until light and fluffy. Add the eggs and vanilla if you're using and beat until well mixed. Fold in the dry ingredients until well combined.

Line a baking tray or spray with non-stick cooking oil, and drop teaspoons of dough on to it. Bake for 8 minutes in the preheated oven.

Invite your friends round, make coffee, dunk and enjoy!

16. The Pyramid Food Tables

Once you become accustomed to living the Pyramid life-style, you'll soon find you no longer need to check your intake of certain macronutrients. It's just like learning to ride a bike. You'll make one or two mistakes to begin with, but as the days go by, the ride will get smoother and smoother – trust me!

The most important things to remember are:

Always aim to eat 1g of protein per lb of body-weight, con-sumed in reasonably equal portions throughout the day, *not* all in one meal.

Do not exceed the net-carb limit for any given day:

High-carb day: 1g per lb of body-weight
Low-carb day: 0.5g per lb of body-weight
No-carb day: 20g

Most foods listed in the tables below are Pyramid-approved. If you can't find what you're looking for, it is probably either high GI/GL, or contains too much fat, sugar or salt. Of course there are foods I haven't listed which common sense will tell you are fine to eat. In these instances, simply compare them with a similar food that is listed.

Processed foods have no place in these tables, and the same goes for products containing additives. Your new-found appreciation for dishes made from only natural ingredients means you will enjoy an enormous variety of satiating flavours without craving junk.

Read these tables before cooking, to help your daily calculations. Please be aware that dried or canned foods may have different properties to their fresh equivalents and are to be avoided unless listed as approved. And always check the labels for manufactured products such as yoghurt, as nutritional data will vary between brands.

Do not consume any non-approved food under any circumstances. A selection of these foods are included in the tables for the avoidance of doubt only because they are often foods you may assume are OK, but in fact are not. For example, parsnips, potatoes and swedes are high GI, but sweet potatoes and yams are medium GI and are therefore the only foods in this group that have made it on to the ticklist.

You'll notice a handful of items are shown as being low GI, yet fall under the non-approved category. They are banned for a reason, so please don't be tempted! These foods are either processed, high in bad fats or salt or full of empty calories. You will also find some popular dishes listed from a variety of different cuisines. Not all of these are approved and are listed to assist you in making the right choices, both in restaurants and when cooking at home.

You'll also notice that a very small number of foods (such as raisins) are marked with an asterisk. These are high GI or high GL, yet still Pyramid-approved as long as they are consumed in moderation and with low GI foods to lower the overall GL of the meal.

These tables are intended as an approximate guide and are not exact. Some figures are rounded up or down for easy calculation and statistics may vary slightly from those quoted previously; this is to reflect a broad range of opinions and food manufacturers.

A–Z of Pyramid-Approved Foods

FRUIT

Food	Quantity	Net Carbs	Protein	Fat	GI	GL	Pyramid-Approved?
Apple	1 medium	9g	0g	0g	L	L	Yes
Apricot	1 medium	4.5g	1g	0g	M	M	Yes
Banana	1 medium	25g	1g	1g	M	H	Yes
Blackberries	100g	2g	1g	0g	L	L	Yes
Blackcurrants	100g	3g	1g	0g	L	L	Yes
Blueberries	70g	7g	0.5g	0g	L	L	Yes
Cantaloupe melon	150g	4.5g	1g	0g	H	H	No
Cherries	100g	10g	1g	0g	L	L	Yes
Clementine	60g	4g	1g	0g	L	L	Yes
Cranberries	75g	0.5g	0g	0g	L	L	Yes
Dates	100g	30g	2g	0g	H	H	No
Figs, fresh	50g	4g	1g	1g	L	L	Yes
Gooseberries	100g	6g	1g	1g	L	L	Yes
Grapefruit	200g	12g	2g	0g	L	L	Yes
Grapes	100g	14g	0g	0g	L	L	Yes
Greengages	100g	8g	1g	0g	L	L	Yes
Guavas	100g	1g	1g	0g	L	L	Yes
Honeydew melon	200g	12g	1g	0g	H	M	Yes

267

Food	Quantity	Net Carbs	Protein	Fat	GI	GL	Pyramid-Approved?
Kiwi Fruit	60g	5g	1g	0g	L	L	Yes
Kumquats	10g	1g	0g	0g	L	L	Yes
Lemons	60g	0g	0g	0g	L	L	Yes
Limes	40g	0g	0g	0g	L	L	Yes
Lychees	90g	12g	1g	0g	L	L	Yes
Mandarin oranges	70g	5.5g	0.5g	0g	L	L	Yes
Mangoes	150g	17g	1g	0g	L	L	Yes
Nectarines	150g	12g	2g	0g	L	L	Yes
Oranges	150g	11g	2g	0g	L	L	Yes
Papayas	150g	9g	1g	0g	M	L	Yes
Passionfruit	60g	1g	2g	0g	L	L	Yes
Peaches	100g	6g	1g	0g	L	L	Yes
Pears	150g	9g	1g	0g	L	L	Yes
Pineapple	80g	7g	0g	0g	M	L	Yes
Plums	50g	4g	0g	0g	L	L	Yes
Pomegranate	50g	4g	1g	0g	L	L	Yes
Prunes	60g	18g	2g	0g	M	L	Yes
Raisins*	30g	20g	1g	0g	M	H	Yes
Raspberries	60g	1.5g	1g	0g	L	L	Yes
Redcurrants	100g	1g	1g	0g	L	L	Yes
Rhubarb	140g	0g	1g	0g	L	L	Yes
Satsumas	70g	5g	1g	0g	L	L	Yes
Starfruit	120g	7g	1g	0g	L	L	Yes
Strawberries	100g	5g	1g	0g	L	L	Yes
Sultanas*	20g	12g	0g	0g	M	H	Yes
Tangerines	70g	5g	1g	0g	L	L	Yes
Watermelon	200g	14g	1g	0g	H	L	Yes

VEGETABLES AND SALAD

Food	Quantity	Net Carbs	Protein	Fat	GI	GL	Pyramid-Approved?
Artichoke	50g	3g	1g	0g	L	L	Yes
Asparagus	125g	0g	4g	1g	L	L	Yes
Aubergine	100g	1g	1g	0g	L	L	Yes
Avocado	100g	1.5g	2g	20g	L	L	Yes
Bamboo shoots	50g	0g	1g	1g	L	L	Yes
Beetroot	40g	3g	1g	0g	M	L	Yes
Blackeye beans	60g	10g	5g	1g	L	M	Yes
Broad beans	120g	0.5g	6g	1g	H	L	Yes
Broccoli	100g	0g	3.5g	1g	L	L	Yes
Brussels sprouts	100g	0g	3g	1g	L	L	Yes
Butter beans	60g	8g	4g	1g	L	L	Yes
Butternut squash	65g	4g	1g	0g	L	L	Yes
Cabbage (red)	90g	0g	1g	0g	L	L	Yes
Cabbage (white)	100g	0.5g	1g	0g	L	L	Yes
Carrots	80g	4g	0g	1g	M	L	Yes
Cauliflower	90g	0.5g	3g	1g	L	L	Yes
Celeriac	30g	0g	0g	0g	L	L	Yes
Celery	30g	0g	0g	0g	L	L	Yes
Chard (swiss)	90g	1g	2g	0g	L	L	Yes
Chickpeas	70g	9g	5g	1g	L	L	Yes
Chicory	30g	1g	0g	1g	L	L	Yes
Chilli pepper (red)	10g	0g	0g	0g	L	L	Yes
Corn-on-the-cob	200g	20g	5g	3g	M	M	Yes
Courgette	90g	1g	2g	1g	L	L	Yes
Cress	5g	0g	0g	0g	L	L	Yes
Cucumber	25g	0g	0g	0g	L	L	Yes
Curly kale	100g	0g	2g	1g	L	L	Yes

Food	Quantity	Net Carbs	Protein	Fat	GI	GL	Pyramid-Approved?
Endive	30g	0g	1g	0g	L	L	Yes
Fennel	40g	1g	0g	0g	L	L	Yes
Garlic	3g	0g	0g	0g	L	L	Yes
Green beans	90g	1g	2g	1g	L	L	Yes
Leek	75g	0.5g	1g	1g	L	L	Yes
Lentils	80g	11g	7g	1g	L	L	Yes
Lettuce (cos)	80g	0g	1g	1g	L	L	Yes
Lettuce (iceberg)	80g	1.5g	1g	0g	L	L	Yes
Mangetout	80g	1.5g	3g	0g	L	L	Yes
Marrow	65g	0.5g	0g	0g	L	L	Yes
Mixed frozen veg	90g	3g	3g	0g	L	L	Yes
Mushrooms	40g	0g	1g	0g	L	L	Yes
Okra	30g	0g	1g	1g	L	L	Yes
Onion	100g	8g	2g	0g	L	L	Yes
Parsnip	65g	5g	1g	1g	H	M	No
Peas	70g	4g	4g	1g	M	L	Yes
Pepper (green)	160g	1.5g	1g	1g	L	L	Yes
Pepper (red)	160g	7.5g	2g	1g	L	L	Yes
Pepper (yellow)	160g	5g	2g	0g	L	L	Yes
Plantain	200g	54g	2g	1g	L	M	Yes
Potato	180g	52g	7g	0g	H	M	No
Pumpkin	60g	0.5g	0g	1g	H	L	Yes
Radishes	50g	0.5g	1g	0g	L	L	Yes
Spinach	90g	0g	3g	0g	L	L	Yes
Spring greens	95g	0g	2g	1g	L	L	Yes
Spring onions	10g	0g	0g	0g	L	L	Yes
Squash	65g	4g	1g	0g	M	L	Yes
Swede	60g	0.5g	0g	0g	H	L	Yes
Sweet potato	130g	25g	1g	1g	L	M	Yes
Sweetcorn	100g	20g	2g	1g	M	M	Yes

Food	Quantity	Net Carbs	Protein	Fat	GI	GL	Pyramid-Approved?
Tomato	85g	2g	1g	1g	L	L	Yes
Turnip	60g	0g	0g	1g	L	L	Yes
Water chestnuts	30g	1g	0g	0g	L	L	Yes
Watercress	20g	0g	1g	1g	L	L	Yes
Yam	130g	40g	2g	1g	L	M	Yes

MEAT

Beef	Quantity	Net Carbs	Protein	Fat	GI	GL	Pyramid-Approved?
Braising steak	100g	0g	30g	10g	M	L	Yes
Fillet steak	100g	0g	30g	6g	M	L	Yes
Flank	100g	0g	30g	15g	M	L	Yes
Mince, lean	100g	0g	23g	4g	M	L	Yes
Ribs	100g	0g	33g	11g	M	L	Yes
Rump steak	100g	0g	30g	10g	M	L	Yes
Silverside	100g	0g	32g	7g	M	L	Yes
Sirloin	100g	0g	32g	6g	M	L	Yes
Stewing steak	100g	0g	29g	6g	M	L	Yes
Topside	100g	0g	33g	9g	M	L	Yes
Chicken	Quantity	Net Carbs	Protein	Fat	GI	GL	Pyramid-Approved?
Breast	100g	0g	24.5g	2g	L	L	Yes
Dark meat	100g	0g	24g	11g	L	L	Yes
Drumsticks	100g	0g	24g	8g	L	L	Yes
Leg	100g	0g	21g	12g	L	L	Yes
Light meat	100g	0g	30g	4g	L	L	Yes
Thigh	100g	0g	20g	14g	L	L	Yes
Wings	100g	0g	27g	17g	L	L	Yes

Lamb	Quantity	Net Carbs	Protein	Fat	GI	GL	Pyramid-Approved?
Breast	100g	0g	25g	15g	M	L	Yes
Chops	100g	0g	25g	12g	M	L	Yes
Cutlet	100g	0g	28g	14g	M	L	Yes
Leg	100g	0g	28g	9g	M	L	Yes
Loin	100g	0g	25g	18g	M	L	Yes
Mince	100g	0g	23g	12g	M	L	Yes
Rack	100g	0g	25g	13g	M	L	Yes
Shoulder	100g	0g	25g	14g	M	L	Yes
Stewing	100g	0g	26g	15g	M	L	Yes
Pork	Quantity	Net Carbs	Protein	Fat	GI	GL	Pyramid-Approved?
Steak	100g	0g	25g	4g	M	L	Yes
Chop	100g	0g	22g	15g	M	L	Yes
Crackling	100g	0g	30g	46g	M	L	No
Fillet	100g	0g	30g	4g	M	L	Yes
Spare rib	100g	0g	23g	10g	M	L	Yes
Bacon (grilled)	100g	0g	26g	12g	M	L	Yes
Gammon joint	100g	0g	25g	13g	M	L	Yes
Gammon rashers (grilled)	100g	0g	28g	10g	M	L	Yes
Ham (sliced)	100g	0g	24g	6g	M	L	Yes
Ham (parma)	100g	0g	26g	6g	M	L	Yes
Turkey & Game	Quantity	Net Carbs	Protein	Fat	GI	GL	Pyramid-Approved?
Turkey breast	100g	0g	25.7g	1.1g	L	L	Yes
Pheasant	100g	0g	25.7g	0.6g	L	L	Yes
Duck	100g	0g	19.9g	4.3g	L	L	Yes
Venison	100g	0g	23.7g	1.4g	L	L	Yes
Rabbit	100g	0g	21.8g	2.4g	L	L	Yes

FISH AND SHELLFISH

Food	Quantity	Net Carbs	Protein	Fat	GI	GL	Pyramid-Approved?
Anchovies	100g	0g	30g	20g	L	L	Yes
Bass	100g	0g	19g	2g	L	L	Yes
Cockles	100g	0g	12g	4g	L	L	Yes
Cod, baked	100g	0g	22g	1g	L	L	Yes
Crab	100g	0g	16g	1.5g	L	L	Yes
Crabsticks	100g	0g	7g	0g	M	L	Yes
Eel, jellied	100g	0g	7g	6g	L	L	Yes
Haddock	100g	0g	25g	1g	L	L	Yes
Halibut	100g	0g	24g	2g	L	L	Yes
Herring	100g	0g	20g	10g	L	L	Yes
John Dory	100g	0g	20.5g	0.5g	L	L	Yes
Kipper	100g	0g	20g	18g	L	L	Yes
Lemon sole	100g	0g	20g	2g	L	L	Yes
Lobster	100g	0g	22g	2g	L	L	Yes
Mackerel	100g	0g	20g	16g	L	L	Yes
Mahi-mahi	100g	0g	18g	1g	L	L	Yes
Monkfish	100g	0g	10g	0g	L	L	Yes
Mullet, grey	100g	0g	26g	5g	L	L	Yes
Mussels	100g	0g	16.5g	2.5g	L	L	Yes
Pilchards	100g	0g	17g	8g	L	L	Yes
Plaice	100g	0g	18g	2g	L	L	Yes
Pollock	100g	0g	18g	2g	L	L	Yes
Prawns	100g	0g	25g	2g	L	L	Yes
Red snapper	100g	0g	23g	3g	L	L	Yes
Roe (cod)	100g	0g	23g	4g	L	L	Yes
Roe (herring)	100g	0g	24g	4g	L	L	Yes
Salmon	100g	0g	20g	11g	L	L	Yes

Food	Quantity	Net Carbs	Protein	Fat	GI	GL	Pyramid-Approved?
Sardines	100g	0g	21g	10g	L	L	Yes
Scallops	100g	2.5g	18g	1.5g	L	L	Yes
Skate	100g	0g	20g	0.5g	L	L	Yes
Sole	100g	0g	17.5g	2g	L	L	Yes
Sprats	100g	0g	25g	15g	L	L	Yes
Squid	100g	0g	13g	1.5g	L	L	Yes
Swordfish	100g	0g	24g	5g	L	L	Yes
Tilapia	100g	0g	21g	0g	L	L	Yes
Trout	100g	0g	22g	6g	L	L	Yes
Tuna	100g	0g	23g	4g	L	L	Yes
Whelks	100g	0g	19g	3.5g	L	L	Yes
Whitebait	100g	0g	18g	5g	L	L	Yes
Whiting	100g	0g	18g	1g	L	L	Yes
Winkles	100g	0g	16g	3.5g	L	L	Yes
Yellowtail snapper	100g	0g	23g	2g	L	L	Yes

DAIRY PRODUCTS

Food	Quantity	Net Carbs	Protein	Fat	GI	GL	Pyramid-Approved?
Brie	40g	2g	8g	12g	L	L	No
Camembert	40g	0g	9g	9g	L	L	No
Cheddar	40g	0g	10g	14g	L	L	No
Cheddar (low-fat)	40g	0g	13g	6g	L	L	Yes
Cheshire	40g	0g	9g	13g	L	L	No
Cottage cheese	40g	0g	5g	2g	L	L	Yes
Cottage cheese (low-fat)	40g	0g	5g	1g	L	L	Yes
Cow's milk (skimmed)	146ml	7g	5g	1g	L	L	Yes
Cow's milk (semi-skimmed)	146ml	7g	5g	2g	L	L	No

Food	Quantity	Net Carbs	Protein	Fat	GI	GL	Pyramid-Approved?
Cow's milk (whole)	146ml	7g	5g	6g	L	L	No
Cream cheese	30g	1g	2.5g	10g	L	L	No
Cream cheese (fat free)	30g	1.5g	4g	0g	L	L	Yes
Cream (clotted)	45g	1g	1g	29g	L	L	No
Cream (double)	30ml	1g	1g	16g	L	L	No
Cream (half)	30ml	1g	1g	4g	L	L	No
Cream (single)	15ml	1g	0g	3g	L	L	No
Crème fraiche	50g	1.5g	1g	20g	L	L	No
Danish blue	30g	0g	6g	9g	L	L	No
Edam	40g	0g	0g	10g	L	L	No
Egg white	32g	0g	3g	0g	L	L	Yes
Egg yolk	18g	0g	3g	1.5g	L	L	Yes
Emmental	40g	0g	12g	12g	L	L	No
Feta	55g	0.5g	8.5g	11g	L	L	No
Fromage frais	100g	17g	5g	5.5g	L	L	No
Goat's milk	55ml	0g	12g	14g	L	L	Yes
Gouda	40g	0g	10g	12g	L	L	No
Mascarpone	55g	0g	3g	24	L	L	No
Mozzarella	55g	0g	14g	11g	L	L	Yes
Parmesan	20g	0g	9g	7g	L	L	No
Parmesan (low-fat)	28g	1.1g	10.5g	7.5g	L	L	Yes
Red leicester	40g	0g	10g	13g	L	L	No
Ricotta	55g	1g	5g	6g	L	L	No
Sheep's milk	146ml	7g	8g	8g	L	L	Yes
Soya milk (unsweetened)	146ml	7g	5g	1g	L	L	Yes
Yoghurt (fruit, no added sugar)	125g	7g	8g	1g	L	L	Yes
Yoghurt (sugar-free Greek style, low-fat)	125g	7g	8g	1g	L	L	Yes
Yoghurt (natural)	125g	8g	6g	1.5g	L	L	Yes
Yoghurt (soya)	125g	12g	3g	2.5g	L	L	Yes

RICE, PASTA AND NOODLES

Food	Quantity	Net Carbs	Protein	Fat	GI	GL	Pyramid-Approved?
Fettucine	100g	18g	3g	0.5g	L	L	No
Gluten-free pasta (brown)	100g	81g	3g	1g	M	M	Yes
Macaroni	100g	20g	4g	1g	M	M	No
Noodles, egg	100g	17g	2g	1g	M	M	No
Rice, basmati	100g	26g	2.5g	0.5g	M	H	No
Rice, brown	100g	30g	2.5g	1g	M	M	Yes
Rice, jasmine	100g	28g	3g	0.5g	H	H	No
Rice, white	100g	28g	3g	1g	M	H	No
Spaghetti (white)	100g	22g	3g	1g	M	M	No
Spaghetti (wholewheat)	100g	30g	5g	1g	L	L	Yes

BREADS AND FLOURS

Food	Quantity	Net Carbs	Protein	Fat	GI	GL	Pyramid-Approved?
Bagel	1 medium	39g	7g	2g	H	H	No
Bread (granary)	1 medium slice	12.5g	3g	1g	L	L	Yes
Bread (soya)	1 medium slice	11g	6g	2g	L	L	Yes
Bread (white)	1 medium slice	16g	3g	1g	H	M	No
Bread (wholemeal)	1 medium slice	13g	3g	1g	M	M	Yes
Chapati (white)	1 medium	75g	10g	1g	M	L	No
Chapati (brown)	1 medium	68g	12g	1g	M	L	Yes
Croissant	1 medium	25g	5g	12g	M	H	No
Flour, white	100g	75g	9g	1g	M	L	No
Flour, brown	100g	55g	13g	2g	M	L	Yes
Flour, soy	100g	28g	49g	1g	L	L	Yes

Food	Quantity	Net Carbs	Protein	Fat	GI	GL	Pyramid-Approved?
French baguette (white)	1 small	29g	5g	0.5g	H	M	No
Garlic bread	3 slices	8g	5g	12g	H	M	No
Naan bread	160g	75g	12g	12g	M	H	No
Pitta bread (white)	75g	39g	7g	1g	M	L	No
Pitta bread (brown)	75g	39g	7g	1g	L	L	Yes
Rolls (granary)	56g	22g	6g	2g	L	L	Yes
Rolls (white)	45g	22g	4g	1g	H	M	No
Rolls (wholemeal)	50g	20g	5g	2g	H	M	Yes
Rye bread	45g	19g	3g	1g	M	L	Yes
Scones	50g	25g	3g	7g	H	H	No
Tortilla wrap (white)	1 wrap	25g	4g	3g	M	M	No
Tortilla wrap (wholemeal)	1 wrap	33g	6g	5g	L	L	Yes
Waffles	65g	25g	6g	11g	M	H	No

BREAKFAST CEREALS

Food	Quantity	Net Carbs	Protein	Fat	GI	GL	Pyramid-Approved?
Bran flakes	30g	17g	3g	1g	H	M	No
Bran strands	40g	9g	6g	1g	L	L	Yes
Clusters (crunchy, with fruit)	50g	19g	4g	5g	H	H	No
Cornflakes	30g	25g	2g	0g	H	H	No
Hoops (honey or nut)	30g	22g	2g	1g	H	H	No
Muesli (no added sugar)	50g	30g	5g	4g	L	L	Yes
Oatbran	1 cup	25g	7g	2g	L	L	Yes
Oatmeal	30g	20g	2g	1g	L	L	Yes

Food	Quantity	Net Carbs	Protein	Fat	GI	GL	Pyramid-Approved?
Porridge, instant, with skimmed milk	40g	20g	8g	5g	L	L	Yes
Porridge, instant, with water	40g	17.5g	8g	14g	M	M	Yes
Porridge oats with water	40g	12g	2g	2g	L	L	Yes
Porridge oats with skimmed milk	40g	21g	8g	5g	L	L	Yes
Puffed rice	30g	12g	3g	0g	H	H	No
Puffed wheat	30g	17g	3g	0g	H	H	No
Shredded wheat	45g	25g	5g	1g	M	M	Yes
Wholewheat biscuits	20g	13g	2g	0g	H	H	No

NUTS AND SNACKS

Food	Quantity	Net Carbs	Protein	Fat	GI	GL	Pyramid-Approved?
Almonds	25g	0g	6g	14g	L	L	Yes
Apricots, dried	120g	36g	5g	1g	L	L	Yes
Bombay mix	30g	9g	6g	10g	M	M	No
Brazil nuts	30g	0g	3g	21g	L	L	Yes
Breadsticks	30g	19g	4g	4g	M	M	No
Cashew nuts	30g	5g	6g	5g	L	L	Yes
Chestnuts	50g	16g	1g	1g	L	L	Yes
Crackers	14g	10g	1g	2g	M	M	No
Digestives	26g	17g	2g	5g	M	H	No
Hazelnuts	30g	0g	1g	6g	L	L	Yes
Hummus	30g	2g	2g	4g	L	L	Yes
Oatmeal crackers	26g	10g	3g	4g	M	M	Yes
Peanuts	30g	5g	8g	5g	L	L	Yes
Pecan nuts	30g	0.5g	6g	42g	L	L	Yes

Food	Quantity	Net Carbs	Protein	Fat	GI	GL	Pyramid-Approved?
Pine nuts	30g	0g	6g	18g	L	L	Yes
Pistachio nuts	30g	0.5g	1g	6g	L	L	Yes
Popcorn (lightly salted)	75g	36g	5g	32g	L	L	Yes
Popcorn (sweetened)	75g	57g	2g	14g	M	M	No
Pretzels	30g	23g	3g	1g	H	H	No
Pumpkin seeds	16g	1g	4g	7g	L	L	Yes
Raisins*	30g	20g	1g	0g	M	H	Yes
Rice cakes	1 rice cake	6g	1g	0g	H	H	No
Ryvita	50g	35g	4g	1g	M	L	Yes
Seed / nut bar (no fruit)	30g	16g	3g	6g	M	M	Yes
Sesame seeds	12g	0g	2g	7g	L	L	Yes
Tortilla chips	50g	27g	4g	11g	M	M	No
Walnuts	30g	0.5g	3g	14g	L	L	Yes

SAUCES, SPREADS, FATS AND OILS

Food	Quantity	Net Carbs	Protein	Fat	GI	GL	Pyramid-Approved?
Apple sauce (homemade)	20g	3g	0g	0g	L	L	Yes
Barbecue sauce	25g	6g	0g	0g	L	L	No
Brown sauce	20g	5g	0g	0g	L	L	No
Butter	20g	0g	0g	16g	L	L	No
Cashew nut butter	30g	8g	5g	15g	L	L	Yes
Chilli sauce	25g	4g	0g	0g	L	L	No
Chocolate spread	16g	9g	1g	6g	L	L	No
Chutney	33g	16g	0g	0g	M	M	No
Coconut oil	11ml	0g	0g	11g	L	L	Yes
Corn oil	15ml	0g	0g	15g	L	L	No
Custard	120ml	19g	3g	1g	L	L	No
Fish paste	10g	0g	2g	1g	L	L	Yes

Food	Quantity	Net Carbs	Protein	Fat	GI	GL	Pyramid-Approved?
Fish pâté	40g	1g	5g	14g	L	L	Yes
Guacamole	45g	0g	1g	6g	L	L	Yes
Hazelnut oil	10ml	0g	0g	54g	L	L	Yes
Honey	17g	13g	0g	0g	M	L	No
Hummus	100g	14g	9g	8g	L	L	Yes
Jam (fruit)	15g	10g	0g	0g	L	L	No
Lemon curd	15g	9g	0g	1g	L	L	No
Liver pâté	40g	0.6g	5.7g	11g	L	L	Yes
Marmalade	15g	10g	0g	0g	L	L	No
Marmite	8g	1.4g	3g	0g	L	L	Yes
Mayonnaise	30g	1g	0g	23g	L	L	No
Mint sauce	10g	2g	0g	0g	L	L	Yes
Mustard	8g	0g	1g	1g	L	L	Yes
Olive oil	11ml	0g	0g	11g	L	L	Yes
Palm oil	11ml	0g	0g	11g	L	L	No
Peanut butter	25g	4g	6g	12g	L	L	Yes
Rapeseed oil	11ml	0g	0g	11g	L	L	No
Salad cream	20g	3g	0g	6g	L	L	No
Sesame oil	9ml	0g	0g	9g	L	L	Yes
Soy sauce, tamari	18g	1g	2g	0g	L	L	Yes
Soya oil	11ml	0g	0g	11g	L	L	Yes
Sunflower oil	11ml	0g	0g	11g	L	L	Yes
Tomato ketchup	15ml	5g	0.5g	0g	L	L	No
Tomato ketchup, sugar-free	15ml	2.5g	0.5g	0g	L	L	Yes
Treacle	50ml	34g	1g	0g	M	L	No
Vegetable oil	11ml	0g	0g	11g	L	L	Yes
Vegetable pâté	80g	3g	6g	11g	L	L	Yes
Walnut oil	11ml	0g	0g	11g	L	L	Yes
Wheatgerm oil	11ml	0g	0g	11g	L	L	No
Yeast extract	9g	0g	4g	0g	L	L	Yes

NON-ALCOHOLIC DRINKS

Drink	Quantity	Net Carbs	Protein	Fat	GI	GL	Pyramid-Approved?
Apple juice	160ml	16g	0g	0g	M	M	No
Cappuccino	190ml	5g	3g	2g	H	H	No
Carrot juice	160ml	9g	1g	0g	L	L	Yes
Chocolate milk	250ml	27g	9g	5g	H	H	No
Coffee	190ml	1g	1g	0g	L	L	Yes
Cola	160ml	17g	0g	0g	M	H	No
Cola (diet)	160ml	0g	0g	0g	L	L	No
Cranberry juice	250ml	36g	0g	0g	M	M	No
Drinking yoghurt	200ml	26g	6g	0g	L	L	No
Fruit juice	200ml	20g	0g	0g	M	M	No
Fruit squash	250ml	9g	0g	0g	M	M	No
Ginger ale	160ml	6g	0g	0g	L	L	No
Grape juice	160ml	19g	0g	0g	L	M	No
Hot chocolate	190ml	20g	6g	8g	H	H	No
Latte (skinny)	190ml	5g	3g	1g	L	L	Yes
Lemonade	160ml	9g	0g	0g	M	H	No
Lemon juice, fresh	100ml	0g	0g	0g	L	L	Yes
Mango juice	160ml	16g	0g	0g	M	H	No
Orange juice	160ml	14g	1g	0g	L	M	No
Ovaltine	190ml	25g	7g	3g	H	H	No
Passionfruit juice	160ml	17g	1g	0g	L	M	No
Pineapple juice	160ml	17g	0g	0g	L	M	No
Sparkling water	200ml	0g	0g	0g	L	L	Yes
Tea, black or green	190ml	0g	0g	0g	L	L	Yes
Tomato juice	160ml	5g	1g	0g	L	L	Yes
Tonic water	160ml	14g	0g	0g	L	L	No

ALCOHOLIC DRINKS

Drink	Quantity	Net Carbs	Protein	Fat	GI	GL	Pyramid-Approved?
Advocat	25ml	7g	1g	2g	M	M	No
Bitter	287ml	6g	1g	0g	H	H	No
Brandy	25ml	0g	0g	0g	L	L	Yes
Brown ale	250ml	8g	1g	0g	H	H	No
Champagne	125ml	2g	0g	0g	L	L	Yes
Cherry brandy	25ml	8g	0g	0g	H	H	No
Cider	287ml	7g	0g	0g	L	L	No
Cointreau	25ml	6g	0g	0g	H	H	No
Cream liqueur	25ml	6g	0g	4g	H	H	No
Curacao	25ml	7g	0g	0g	H	H	No
Egg nog	160ml	16g	6g	7g	H	H	No
Gin	25ml	0g	0g	0g	L	L	Yes
Guinness	287ml	4g	1g	0g	H	H	No
Lager	250ml	4g	1g	0g	H	H	No
Mulled wine	125ml	32g	0g	0g	L	L	No
Port	50ml	6g	0g	0g	L	L	Yes
Red wine	125ml	3g	0g	0g	L	L	Yes
Rosé wine	125ml	3g	0g	0g	L	L	Yes
Rum	25ml	0g	0g	0g	L	L	Yes
Sherry	50ml	3g	0g	0g	L	L	Yes
Vermouth, dry	50ml	1g	0g	0g	L	L	Yes
Vodka	25ml	0g	0g	0g	L	L	Yes
Whisky	25ml	0g	0g	0g	L	L	Yes
White wine (dry)	125ml	3g	0g	0g	L	L	Yes
White wine (medium)	125ml	4g	0g	0g	L	L	Yes
White wine (sweet)	125ml	7g	0g	0g	L	L	No

Restaurant Dishes

CHINESE AND ORIENTAL FOOD

Food	Quantity	Net Carbs	Protein	Fat	GI	GL	Pyramid-Approved?
Aromatic crispy duck	125g	14g	35g	30g	L	L	Yes
Beef chow mein	350g	42g	30g	32g	M	H	No
Beef in black bean sauce	360g	4g	38g	20g	L	L	Yes
Beef stir-fry (cashew)	350g	18.5g	36g	39g	L	L	Yes
Chicken balls	4 balls	11g	15g	11g	M	M	No
Chicken chop suey	250g	4g	18g	10g	L	L	Yes
Chicken chow mein	350g	42g	28g	25g	M	H	No
Chicken in black bean sauce	350g	10g	25g	28g	L	L	Yes
Chicken satay	1 skewer	3g	22.5g	5g	L	L	Yes
Chicken stir-fry	350g	2g	24g	14g	L	L	Yes
Chicken with cashew nuts	360g	40g	24g	39g	L	L	Yes
Clear soups	55g	10g	4g	3g	L	L	Yes
Curried beef	100g	28g	28g	18g	L	L	Yes
Curried chicken (green Thai)	350g	0g	31g	30g	L	L	Yes
Curried pork	150g	3g	28g	22g	L	L	Yes
Egg-fried rice	270g	85g	12g	13g	M	H	No
Mussels in black bean sauce	250g	16g	31g	9g	L	L	Yes
Pancakes	70g	37g	6g	6g	M	H	No
Pork chow mein	350g	46g	24g	14g	M	M	No
Pork in black bean sauce	350g	4g	36g	22g	M	M	Yes
Pork satay	1 skewer	3g	24g	6g	L	L	Yes
Prawn crackers	70g	36g	0g	27g	L	M	No
Prawn sesame toast	70g	11g	9g	21g	M	M	No
Singapore noodles	250g	54g	9g	12g	M	M	No
Spare ribs (dry)	340g	6g	75g	64g	L	L	Yes
Spring rolls	55g	9g	4g	9g	M	M	No

Food	Quantity	Net Carbs	Protein	Fat	GI	GL	Pyramid-Approved?
Steamed fish	100g	0g	24g	3g	L	L	Yes
Steamed rice	132g	45g	4g	0g	M	M	No
Steamed tofu	84g	2g	6g	2g	L	L	Yes
Steamed veg	150g	4.4g	2g	0g	L	L	Yes
Stir-fried vegetables	340g	1g	6g	14g	L	L	Yes
Sweet and sour chicken	300g	56g	23g	30g	L	L	No
Sweet and sour pork (battered)	300g	60g	23g	42g	L	L	No
Szechuan prawns with veg	350g	6g	27g	16g	L	L	Yes

INDIAN FOOD

Food	Quantity	Net Carbs	Protein	Fat	GI	GL	Pyramid-Approved?
Beef madras	350g	6g	32g	29g	L	L	Yes
Bombay potatoes	159g	12.5g	2g	6.5g	H	H	No
Chapati	110g	75g	10g	1g	M	L	No
Chicken biryani	400g	62g	34g	30g	M	M	No
Chicken jalfrezi	350g	4g	34g	27g	L	L	Yes
Chicken korma	350g	1g	44g	51g	L	L	No
Chicken madras	350g	6g	38g	26g	L	L	No
Chicken tikka	350g	0g	65g	15g	L	L	Yes
Chicken tikka masala	350g	10g	40g	40g	L	L	No
King prawn bhuna	350g	8g	29g	30g	L	L	Yes
Lamb balti	350g	4g	11g	35g	L	L	Yes
Lamb madras	350g	6g	28g	35g	L	L	Yes
Lamb rogan josh	350g	3g	43g	35g	L	L	No
Meat samosas	70g	11.5g	8g	12g	L	L	No
Naan bread	160g	77g	12g	12g	M	M	No

Food	Quantity	Net Carbs	Protein	Fat	GI	GL	Pyramid-Approved?
Onion bhaji	50g	8g	2g	6g	M	L	No
Poppadoms	70g	16g	8g	27g	H	H	No
Prawn bhuna	400g	0g	6g	35g	L	L	No
Prawn madras	350g	1g	27g	29g	L	L	No
Sag aloo	260g	18g	6g	18g	H	M	No
Sweet mango chutney	33g	16g	0g	0g	H	H	No
Tandoori chicken	350g	48g	35g	3g	L	L	No
Vegetable balti	350g	16g	8g	28g	L	L	Yes
Vegetable biryani	350g	49g	10g	25g	M	M	No
Vindaloo	320g	45g	16g	3.5g	L	L	Yes

MEDITERRANEAN FOOD

Food	Quantity	Net Carbs	Protein	Fat	GI	GL	Pyramid-Approved?
Beef carpaccio	78g	7g	15g	12g	L	L	Yes
Bruschetta	1 piece	1.5g	1.5g	4g	M	M	No
Calzone (meat)	1 calzone	67g	28g	30.5g	H	H	No
Calzone (vegetable)	1 calzone	67g	0g	30.5g	H	H	No
Cannelloni (meat)	400g	42g	24g	26g	H	M	No
Cannelloni (vegetable)	400g	69g	21g	21g	H	M	No
Carbonara	237g	47g	21g	14g	M	M	No
Deep-fried calamari	170g	16g	30g	10g	H	M	No
Fettuccine	100g	18g	3g	0.5g	L	L	No
Gamberoni Pil Pil	132g	2g	14g	12g	L	L	Yes
Garlic bread	3 slices	21g	5g	12g	H	M	No
Goat's cheese salad	1 medium	32g	18g	14g	L	L	Yes
Lasagne	420g	63g	31g	26g	H	H	No
Lasagne (vegetarian)	420g	48g	17g	19g	H	H	No

Food	Quantity	Net Carbs	Protein	Fat	GI	GL	Pyramid-Approved?
Meatballs	100g	0g	25g	17g	L	L	Yes
Minestrone	240g	12g	4.5g	2g	M	L	Yes
Mozzarella & tomato salad	125g	3g	13g	8g	L	L	Yes
Parma ham	40g	0g	8g	8g	L	L	Yes
Parma ham with melon	240g	12g	9g	1g	M	M	Yes
Penne	100g	22g	3g	1g	M	M	No
Penne (wholewheat)	100g	16g	5g	1g	L	L	Yes
Pizza (meat)	115g slice	30g	14g	13g	M	M	No
Pizza (vegetarian)	115g slice	30g	6g	9g	M	M	No
Ravioli	200g	46g	15g	10g	M	M	No
Risotto (plain)	290g	59g	12g	19g	H	H	No
Risotto (chicken)	340g	84g	31g	10g	H	H	No
Scallops	100g	2.5g	18g	1.5g	L	L	Yes
Scampi	170g	35g	16g	23g	M	M	No
Spaghetti bolognese	200g	22g	18g	12g	M	M	No
Spaghetti bolognese (wholemeal)	200g	16g	18g	12g	L	L	Yes
Spaghetti (white)	100g	22g	3g	1g	M	M	No
Spaghetti (wholemeal)	100g	16g	5g	1g	L	L	Yes
Tuna niçoise	medium	15g	19g	5g	L	L	Yes
Veal escalope	1 serving	0g	26g	2g	L	L	Yes

BRITISH FOOD

Food	Quantity	Net Carbs	Protein	Fat	GI	GL	Pyramid-Approved?
Apple crumble	100g	33g	2g	4g	M	M	No
Apple pie	100g	42g	4g	12g	M	M	No
Baked potato	180g	52g	7g	0g	H	M	No

Food	Quantity	Net Carbs	Protein	Fat	GI	GL	Pyramid-Approved?
Beef stew	280g	12g	34g	14g	M	L	Yes
Blackberry crumble	100g	33g	2g	4g	M	M	No
Boiled eggs	2 eggs	0g	12g	3g	L	L	Yes
Cheeseburger	1 burger	28g	20g	14g	H	H	No
Chicken burger	1 burger	42.5g	39.5g	23.5g	H	H	No
Chicken casserole	260g	7g	33g	5g	L	L	No
Chicken drumstick (no skin)	45g	0g	12g	4g	L	L	Yes
Chicken kiev	170g	18g	32g	29g	H	H	No
Chicken & leek soup	100g	3.7g	2.4g	2g	L	L	Yes
Chicken & mushroom pie	100g	14g	13g	10g	H	H	No
Chilli con carne (brown rice)	120g	15g	8g	5g	L	L	Yes
Chips	165g	52g	6g	17g	H	H	No
Cod in batter	180g	25g	23g	21g	H	M	No
Corned beef	21g	0g	6g	3g	L	L	Yes
Cornish pasty	155g	41g	10g	28g	M	M	No
Fish fingers	4 fingers	12g	12g	8g	L	L	No
Fish pie	125g	11g	11g	7g	M	M	No
Haggis	105g	40g	22g	46g	M	L	Yes
Hash brown	1 portion	10g	1g	4g	H	H	No
Macaroni cheese	300g	53g	28g	34g	M	M	No
Mashed potato with butter	120g	18g	2g	5g	H	M	No
New potatoes	175g	25g	2g	1g	H	H	No
Omelette	2 egg	0g	12g	5g	L	L	Yes
Onion rings	120g	39g	6g	17g	L	L	No
Poached eggs	2 eggs	0g	12g	3g	L	L	Yes
Potato wedges	180g	52g	7g	0g	H	H	No
Quiche	140g	25g	15g	20g	M	M	No
Quorn	100g	5g	18g	3g	L	L	Yes
Roast potatoes	130g	32g	4g	6g	H	M	No
Sausage roll	60g	15g	6g	17g	M	M	No

Food	Quantity	Net Carbs	Protein	Fat	GI	GL	Pyramid-Approved?
Sausage & mash	3 + 355g mash	73g	31g	53g	H	H	No
Scrambled eggs	2 eggs	0g	14g	3g	L	L	Yes
Shepherd's pie	240g	50g	33g	43g	M	M	No
Steak pie	120g	26g	16g	26g	M	M	No
Stuffing (white bread)	2 balls	13g	2g	1g	L	L	No
Stuffing (brown bread)	2 balls	12g	2g	1g	L	L	Yes
Tofu	84g	2g	6g	2g	L	L	Yes
Tomato soup	135g	10g	1g	5g	L	L	Yes
Vegetable soup	133g	13g	2g	1g	L	L	Yes
Yorkshire pudding	1 pudding	5.5g	1.5g	1.8g	H	H	No

Acknowledgements

I would like to express my deepest gratitude to those, without whom this book would simply not have been possible.

To my mum, Diana, for giving me such a healthy start in life. I could never have done this without you.

To my dad, Robin, for your eternal support. Thank you for believing in me.

To my nan and granddad, thank you for all the wonderfully active holidays we enjoyed.

Finally, I'd like to thank my agent, Rebecca Winfield and my editor, Katy Follain. Rebecca: you are a truly wonderful, uplifting woman, and if I have one person to thank for this book seeing the light of day, it is you. Katy: you are an incredibly patient editor and I could not have worked with a better publishing house.

Further Reading

Books

Anderson, Tracy, *Tracy Anderson's 30-Day Method* (United Kingdom: Vermilion, 2010)

Challem, Jack, Berkson M.D., Berton, and Smith, Melissa Diane, *Syndrome X* (Canada: John Wiley & Sons, Inc. 2000)

Chan, Dr Wynnie, *GI and GL Counter* (United Kingdom: Octopus Publishing Group Ltd, 2006)

Cheyette, Chris and Balolia, Yello, *Carbs and Cals and Protein and Fat* (United Kingdom: Chello Publishing Ltd, 2010)

Courteney, Hazel, *500 of the Most Important Health Tips You'll Ever Need* (London: CICO Books, 2001)

Dukan, Dr Pierre, *The Dukan Diet* (London: Hodder & Stoughton, 2010)

Malkov M.D., Roman, *The Carb Cycling Diet* (New York: Hatherleigh Press, 2005)

Marshall, David, *Bodydoctor* (London: Harper Collins, 2004)

Westman, Dr Eric, Phinney, Dr Stephen, and Volek, Dr Jeff, *New Atkins, New You* (United Kingdom: Vermilion, 2010)

Websites

http://nutrigenie.net/gid/
http://www.food-database.co.uk/
http://nutritiondata.self.com/

http://www.livestrong.com/
http://www.mycoprotein.org/
http://exercise.about.com/
http://www.fatsecret.com/
http://www.netdoctor.co.uk/
http://www.eatwild.com/healthbenefits.htm
http://www.gilisting.com/
http://www.glycemicindex.com/
http://www.omega3-6-9.com/
http://www.carbs-information.com/
http://www.dannifit.com

DANNI LEVY is a 27-year-old health and fitness journalist who has a number of celebrity clients. An expert contributor for *Closer* magazine's diet and fitness pages, she is also a regular contributor for the *Sun, Love It!, Health & Fitness, Bella* magazine, *Body Fit* magazine and other titles. She runs 5 Star Bootcamp, a luxurious Marbella-based health and fitness bootcamp programme, presents a diet and workout show on the Active Channel (SKY 281) and has featured on Living TV's *Bigger Than . . .* series. A popular fitness model, she has appeared on the covers of numerous fitness magazines around the world.

www.dannilevy.com

MIGUEL TORIBIO-MATEUS is a London-based nutritional therapy consultant with two busy clinics in Harley Street and Belsize Park. Born in Spain, Miguel has a love of cooking and a life-long passion for good food. A perpetual student, with numerous degrees under his belt, he is currently a lecturer at the Institute for Optimum Nutrition, where he is part of a research team focusing on stress-related conditions. He has been featured in a series for Sky TV where he acted as nutritional consultant and expert on celebrity diets and weight-loss. His tips on healthy eating are frequently featured on national press and lifestyle magazines. You can follow Miguel on Twitter @naturopatica.

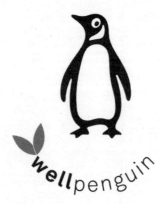

Interested in self help, spiritual and above all inspirational books?

Then join us at

WellPenguin

the exclusive Penguin facebook club for anyone who is curious about life.

- Put questions to our expert authors
- Download free wellbeing podcasts
- Enter our exciting monthly competitions
- Share your views and opinions
- Test yourself with our exclusive quizzes
- Be the first to discover about the next WellPenguin release

www.facebook.com/WellPenguin